A Practical Guide to End of Life Care

A Practical Guide to End of Life Care

Edited by Clair Sadler

 Open University Press

Open University Press
McGraw-Hill Education
McGraw-Hill House
Shoppenhangers Road
Maidenhead
Berkshire
England
SL6 2QL

email: enquiries@openup.co.uk
world wide web: www.openup.co.uk

and Two Penn Plaza, New York, NY 10121-2289, USA

First published 2015

A catalogue record of this book is available from the British Library

ISBN-13: 978-0-335-26356-1
ISBN-10: 0-335-26356-9
eISBN: 978-0-335-26357-8

Library of Congress Cataloging-in-Publication Data
CIP data applied for

Typeset by Transforma Pvt. Ltd., Chennai, India

Fictitious names of companies, products, people, characters and/or data that may
be used herein (in case studies or in examples) are not intended to represent any
real individual, company, product or event.

Printed and bound by CPI Group (UK) Ltd, Croydon, CR0 4YY

Praise for this book

"This is a beautifully presented learning tool to support the delivery of end of life care. I particularly like the 'signposts' which reinforce the intention of the book to enable 'carers' to apply what they read to their role in practice."

Liz Bryan, Director of Education and Training, St Christopher's Hospice, UK

Contents

Foreword

The way people are cared for in their final days and hours lives on in the memory of families for years. I know this as families often remind me years after a loved one has died of a detail of care, such as the way someone was washed, or how some ice cream was tenderly given on a teaspoon.

The *tone* of care, i.e. how care is given, rather than what is done, is crucial to the dignity of those we support. The question has often been asked whether compassion can be taught. I believe care is about kindness and respect for the person and their body rather than simply a set of skills or a particular personality. It is also about confidence and this wise and practical book will give you the confidence and guidance to say and do the right thing and to understand the patient and family journey.

Care is also about teamwork in this day and age – family carers and healthcare support workers sharing the care with specialists, to support people at home, in care homes, in hospital and in hospices. To really feel part of this team, a deeper understanding of the physical and psychological aspects of the dying process will make your contribution so much more valuable.

We know that how the body is treated contributes to the self-esteem of a patient. Our bodies are our most precious possession and when they begin to fail, they need tender care. We also know that the most intimate moments of care often lead to disclosures of fears and worries that are often not revealed to other professional staff. Carers often worry about what to say, when to stay quiet, how to listen, what to share. Again, in this aspect of care, reflecting on the case studies in this book will increase your confidence.

It is this delicate, fragile but vital relationship between carer and patient that this book celebrates and supports.

Dr Ros Taylor, MBE
National Director for Hospice Care
Hospice UK

Contributors

At the time of writing, all the contributors to this book work at Princess Alice Hospice in Esher, Surrey. Princess Alice Hospice offers specialist palliative care to a population of over a million people in Surrey and Middlesex. The in-patient unit has 28 beds offering symptom management, terminal care, psychosocial support, rehabilitation admissions and respite care. As will be seen in this book many people who are approaching the end of their life wish to be cared for in their own homes, including care homes.

The hospice has a community team of over 30 clinical nurse specialists offering care to approximately 800 patients and their families in their own homes. It also provides rapid response, enhanced support and night home care service. There is also a Day Hospice offering day care, therapies, social groups and outpatient services.

The writers of this book all work in a number of different departments and roles within the organisation; however, they have one thing in common and that is a passion to ensure that people approaching the end of their life have the best quality of care, regardless of where they are being cared for.

Jane Berg	Head of Education
Roz Claydon	Staff Nurse
Beverly Clayton	Clinical Nurse Specialist
Karen Cook	Practice Educator
Sue Dunlop	Staff Nurse
Sarah Dowd	Social Worker
Amanda Free	Speciality Doctor
Helen Healey	Staff Nurse
Belinda Hitchens	Occupational Therapist
Christine Linley	Staff Nurse

Hayley Palfreyman	Social Worker
Liz Reed	Research Lead
Clair Sadler	Senior Lecturer
Gill Thomas	Practice Educator
Irene Webster	Staff Nurse

We would also like to acknowledge the contributions of Celia Di Cicco, Vicky Eves, Sue Howard, John Lansdell, Pippa Lee, and Sarah Scoble.

Introduction

Thinking about dying: setting the scene

Jane Berg and Clair Sadler

> You matter because you are you, and you matter to the end of your life. We will do all we can, not only to help you die peacefully, but also to live until you die.
>
> (Dame Cicely Saunders, nurse, physician, writer, and founder of the modern hospice movement, 1918–2005)

If you are reading this book, you are probably involved in the care of people who are facing the end of their life. If you have not been heavily involved in caring for dying people before, the prospect can seem daunting, frightening and a big responsibility. You may be concerned about how to speak to a dying person, what they will expect from you and the kinds of needs they might have. You might also feel concerned about interacting with their family and friends, how they are going to react, what questions might they ask and how will you feel about discussing such things.

In this first chapter we will consider how to use this book and the various activities and case studies you will encounter. The chapter will also encourage you to consider how your views of death may shape the care that you offer others.

How to use this book

This book is a practical guide to help you look after people as they approach the end of their life. It is aimed at anyone who is interested in looking after people as their condition deteriorates and they need more care. The book is based on the view that many people nearing the end of their life do not always need specialist care services. While specialist care services are available and can be very helpful, there are also many things that can be done by non-specialists. This book therefore is aimed at anyone wishing to give the best possible care to someone approaching the end of their life and offers straightforward ideas and practical advice as to how this can be achieved. We may not be able to influence the time of death but we can influence the way in which a person dies and the quality of their death. We can, with understanding and confidence, help a person at this time. As Dame Cicely Saunders said: 'to die peacefully and live until they die'.

Each chapter in this book poses a question and through information, case studies and activities will encourage you to think and understand the many different aspects of end of life care. Physical needs will be discussed alongside the emotional concerns that a person may experience. The importance of communicating will be considered and the services available to help you and the people you care for will be identified. **Chapter 11** is dedicated to ways that may help you as a carer cope with this. At the end of this book you will find a Glossary of some of the words and phrases that you may come across, together with an Appendix giving a list of useful websites and a reading list. The Glossary term is shown in bold on its first occurrence in the chapter. There is also a brief reference list.

There is a strong reflective element to the book, encouraging you to consider what you are learning about, the people that you care for and the situation that you are in.

People providing care may have a variety of job titles and places of work so for the purpose of this book the term 'carer' will be used – simply meaning someone who cares.

The signposts in this book

The reason that many people choose to work in caring roles is often because they are practical people and want to make a difference. One of the best ways to learn is by doing – taking something I'm reading and then applying this learning to my situation. Throughout the book you will see a series of symbols that will be prompts to an activity so that you can apply the knowledge that you have gained to your own unique situation. Each signpost has a different purpose but all are designed to enrich your knowledge of end of life care.

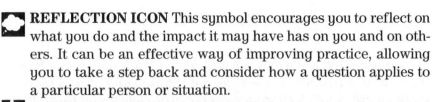 **REFLECTION ICON** This symbol encourages you to reflect on what you do and the impact it may have has on you and on others. It can be an effective way of improving practice, allowing you to take a step back and consider how a question applies to a particular person or situation.

SIGNPOST ICON This symbol will direct you to other related information and resources. Also, at the end of this book in the Appendix, you will find a number of useful resources that you may wish to access. Many of these are websites but you will also find books, DVDs and YouTube clips that will help you care for people at this very significant stage of their life.

FIND OUT ICON The book offers guidance on the information you need to provide quality end of life care; throughout the book you will be encouraged to identify the services and resources in your own specific locality.

PERSON ICON Much of what we learn comes from the people that we care for. Throughout the book there will be extracts from case studies. These are stories, based loosely on real people reaching the end of their lives. The case studies highlight how well people can die with the right support, but also how things can sometimes go wrong.

The stories of three families

In this section we will introduce you to the stories of the three people that we will follow thoughout the book. The people are unique, but their experiences can be transferred to a number of different situations, to different people and to different care settings. In each chapter you will learn a little bit more about them, their families and their experiences, and the things that did and didn't work so well for them.

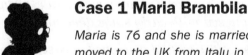 ### Case 1 Maria Brambila

Maria is 76 and she is married to Aldo who is also 76. They moved to the UK from Italy in their early twenties when they were just married and have recently retired from running their family-owned restaurant which is now managed by their two daughters, Lily and Nancy. They have a son, Angelo, who lives in the USA. All three children are married and Maria and Aldo are the proud grandparents to 9 grandchildren, aged between 7 and 21 years.

Maria had her first heart attack at age 65 and has had two more since. After the second heart attack she became breathless and her legs became very swollen. The cardiologist told her she had heart failure.

Six months later, she was visited by her GP after Aldo called him to report that Maria was not eating, not sleeping and feeling increasingly unwell. Maria's GP contacted the cardiologist and was told the treatment options had all been exhausted. The GP visited Maria at home and told her that there was nothing more the hospital could do. Maria and Aldo were adamant that she wanted to die at home, supported by district nurses.

Case 2 Albert Hughes

Albert is 74, a retired carpenter. Albert never married and he lives alone. He has a close circle of 'mates' and a niece, Jackie, who visits regularly. He is a regular at the local bowls club where he enjoys his pipe and a pint and following his favourite football team Arsenal.

When Albert was 71, his friends began to notice he was missing from events at the club, forgetting when they had arranged to meet. They contacted Albert's niece, Jackie, to say they were worried about him.

On her next visit to him, Jackie noticed that Albert had food in the fridge that was mouldy and she suggested to Albert that she should throw it away. He became angry, shouting at her for 'always interfering'. Two months later, the police were called when Albert started to get agitated in the bank when the cashier wouldn't give him any money because he had no cheque book or card. The police returned him home and informed Albert's GP, Dr Evans, that his behaviour was causing concern.

Dr Evans called on Albert and an appointment was made at the memory clinic. He was diagnosed with early stage dementia.

Six months later, as Albert's condition had worsened, a case conference was held with Albert, Jackie, Dr Evans and the social worker. It was discussed that, despite having regular help at home, he was losing weight, finding it difficult to manage the house and garden and that he should move to a care home.

Albert moved to a care home where he quickly settled. After being there for a year, he suddenly became very drowsy and lost the use of his right arm and leg. He was taken to hospital and Jackie was called. He was seen quickly and was diagnosed as having had a stroke.

Jackie was concerned that none of the people caring for him knew what he wanted to happen at the end of his life. Dr Evans, Jackie and Albert's key worker decided to meet with Albert to explore his wishes. Although communication was difficult, with Jackie's support, Albert made it clear he wanted to be cared for in the care home until his death, but did not want any more antibiotics for a chest infection or to be resuscitated if his heart stopped. He had had enough and wanted to die. Dr Evans and the care home documented this as an advance care plan and a Do Not Attempt Cardio Pulmonary Resuscitation (DNACPR) order. Copies of both documents were kept in Albert's care home notes and in his GP notes.

Case 3 Jenny Baxter

Jenny is a 69-year-old retired administrator and has been married to Stephen for 40 years. Jenny and Stephen have two adult children; Sarah, who is married to Dave and has two children, Poppy, 4 years old, and 10-year-old Mark. Their son Andrew is married to Elena, has one son, Ben, aged 11, and they live 200 miles away.

Jenny and Stephen have had a difficult relationship with their daughter-in-law which is a source of great sadness to them as they don't see their son and grandson as much as they would like and the relationships with their son and his family is strained. Jenny's 91-year-old mother Freda is frail and lives in a care home in the same town. Jenny has a good relationship with her mother, she visits her three or four times a week in the care home and, until recently, they have enjoyed regular outings together.

Jenny was diagnosed with advanced breast cancer four years ago, she has had four different cycles of palliative chemotherapy over the past four years which she coped with well. Jenny only recently stopped looking after her grandchildren after school until her daughter, Sarah, came home from work.

Jenny's condition has recently deteriorated; Sarah decided to give up work to help her father take care of her mother.

The stories of Maria, Albert and Jenny will be followed throughout the book. We will now consider how our ideas of death and dying are formed and how this may affect the care that we offer people approaching the end of their lives.

Thinking reflectively about dying

People approach the thought of death and dying in very different ways. It is important to consider how we as individuals approach the end of life and how it makes us feel. This in turn will help us have some understanding of how a dying person and their family might be thinking and how we are best able to support them with empathy and compassion.

Often, we think about what we are doing at that moment without always considering the things that have shaped our thoughts and actions. Throughout this book you will be encouraged to think more deeply about what you do, why you do it that way and the impact this may have. The remainder of this chapter will encourage you to consider how you think about death and dying and how the views of the people we care for are shaped. So to start with, think about if you have ever had a conversation about death or dying. Who was it with? Who started the conversation? How did you feel? What did you discover? How did the conversation end?

The words we use

Such conversations are difficult, especially if our own death seems a very long way off. In our society, the subject of death has been described as the last taboo, a topic that many feel uncomfortable talking about. One sign of our discomfort are the words we use to avoid saying 'death' or 'dying'. Dying Matters, (www.dying-matters.org) is a coalition that through campaigns raises awareness and discussion about dying and bereavement. They suggest that there are over 200 euphemisms, alternative words and phrases that are used. You might have heard that someone has 'lost' a relative, or that someone has 'passed away' or 'passed over'. Here are some other examples:

- gone to meet his maker
- pushing up daisies
- six foot under
- gone to join the angels
- met his maker

- sleeping the big sleep
- popped their clogs
- given up the ghost.

You might want to add to the list with words or phrases that you use or have heard.

Think about why we would want people to feel able to talk about dying. What do you think are the things that make it difficult to discuss dying?

What influences how we think about death?

In the UK, we are living in times of relative peace. We have not experienced large-scale war or conflict in our own country for many decades. This means that most of us have not faced a situation where large numbers of people of the same age as ourselves have died in war or civil conflict.

If you are caring for someone who is elderly, you might want to think about how they experienced the losses in their lives. They may have lived through the Second World War. They may have been in a position where they were themselves at risk of dying young if they were directly involved in the war. It is very likely that they knew of people who died, friends, family or spouse.

In the UK, we have the National Health Service which provides healthcare, health promotion and illness prevention which help us avoid many of the causes of death we would otherwise experience. Consider the experience of people living through epidemics, such as the influenza epidemic in 1918, which killed large numbers of people. Many families would have experienced the death of a member of the family or of people they knew. The illness was very common among young, fit people making it devastating to those who knew them but it also affected the economy of the country with a reduction in the number of people of working age.

However, today we have developed the expectation that doctors can cure most illnesses. We know that new medicines and other treatments are being developed to help us not only with infections, such as mumps and chickenpox and pneumonia, which were the cause of death for many of our grandparents' generation, but also new surgical techniques for heart disease and organ failure. Even dementia, which for so long was seen as almost inevitable in old age, now can be treated to slow down the process of decline. These are positive developments, but bring the expectation that everything can be cured and that death is somehow a failure of the doctors to find the 'right' treatment or to provide it in time.

Of course, not everyone in a country lives in the same way. Your community will also influence your approach to death. A community can be described as a group of people who share a common factor, for instance, a geographical location such as the town or village. A community might also be centred around a shared belief, such as a place of worship, or an interest like a sport or hobby, a specific pub perhaps. It might also be a group of people brought together because of circumstances, such as homelessness or attending a particular school or place of work.

Think about the various communities you are a part of. The community might have specific approaches and rituals associated with death.

Death in a multicultural society

A wide variety of people from different cultures and backgrounds now live in the UK and it is multicultural population, therefore, we will have to care for people from a range of different countries and backgrounds. Some have moved from their country of origin for economic, social or family reasons, but some will have been forced to move because of dangerous situations where they might have felt under threat or may have experienced the death of people from their family or community. There is therefore a richness of ways in which death is experienced and expressed.

Having a different view of rituals around death can influence how we care for people and how we feel about what is 'right'. A district nurse visiting someone in a Traveller family reflected on the fact that she felt uncomfortable delivering care in the presence of the very large extended family who gathered to offer support to the dying person. In her experience, dying was something that is usually attended only by close family members. She found it difficult to know who to talk to, who to share information with. Her feeling of a lack of privacy made her feel so uncomfortable that she found herself not talking to that family in the way she would have done with other non-Traveller families.

The way we behave in relation to dying and death is also influenced by the culture within our own immediate families. Emotions shown and expected vary. There may be a family culture of a 'stiff upper lip' where emotional displays cause embarrassment and discomfort. Other families might share the experience of demonstrating emotions together, with open tears and wailing.

In addition to cultural and religious differences, there are also regional differences. In some parts of the country, for example, it is considered respectful for neighbours and the family of a person who has just died to close the curtains of their house until after the funeral. In some care homes the death of a resident is marked by lighting a candle in a public area. You might notice that these traditions change over time, many of them observed more by the older generations. In some areas it has become common for the death of a person in a road traffic accident to be marked by placing flowers at the roadside where the accident happened, while in some cities white bicycles are placed where a cyclist has died. Increasingly, social media such as Twitter or Facebook are used to mark a person's death. Online fundraising, tribute pages and blogs are other ways in which a person's death may be marked.

In communities there are expectations about how a bereaved person will behave and in some cases how they will look.

The ritual of funerals

Funerals are a significant part of most societies' observance of death. They are a means of publicly acknowledging that a person has died, are a dignified tribute to the life of the person and often a source of comfort to those bereaved to see how others considered and respected their loved one.

There is often an etiquette surrounding a funeral. Wearing black to a funeral, for example, is still considered the usual practice in the UK but the bereaved are no longer expected to continue to wear it for any length of time. White is the traditional colour of mourning for many religions such as Sikhism. Increasingly, however, the person who has died might leave instructions in advance or a family may suggest what mourners wear, specifying bright colours, for example.

Many funerals will follow strict religious observances and have specific rituals related to how long mourning should last and how the body is cared for. The actual funeral service itself may be surrounded by ritual. For example, by tradition, only Muslim men attend the graveside, whereas some communities of African or Caribbean descent may see the internment as a service of thanksgiving for the person's life and will sing and reminisce at the graveside.

Planning a funeral

Increasingly, the funeral service is designed to reflect the interests and beliefs of the person who has died. The music, the coffin and the floral tributes, and the way the ceremony is conducted can be seen as focused on the individual. Many people who know that they are dying take great comfort in planning their own funeral. When caring for someone who is looking ahead and planning their own funeral, it

 is sometimes uncomfortable for carers or family to hear those details. **Chapter 10** offers more information on what happens after someone dies.

How have you felt about funerals you have been involved with or seen on television? Think about the different groups of people you care for in your community, what kind of ceremony is common?

Families and other communities often have an expectation, which is unspoken, of how long it will take for the bereaved person to start to behave 'normally' again and move on from their grief. It is often thought in Western culture that once the funeral is over, things will be better. Other cultures have longer periods of mourning where the bereaved are visited regularly by those in their community. The person who continues to behave as a grieving person for less time or longer than is expected could be a source of concern, impatience or embarrassment for the community.

The public view of death

Large-scale public demonstrations of grief following the death of someone 'famous' seem to have becoming increasingly acceptable in recent years. Their fame may be related to their celebrity status or the manner in which they died. Think, for example, of the public response to the murder of a child, teacher, soldier or police officer. This growth in public outpouring is thought to have started with the death of Princess Diana in 1997 when millions of people were involved in public exhibitions of grief either by adding to the floral tributes formed in public places, or by joining specific gatherings. The public display of tears and anguish was something not seen before in the UK and, as it was broadcast on TV, was shared by many others. For many people watching, the crowd's grief represented the first time it became acceptable to cry in public and this has made open displays of grief about people who have died more common.

Many of our attitudes are formed by the media. We have instant access to world news that is constantly updated, 24 hours a day. The deaths of people from violence or from natural disasters are seen daily on television and computer screens. The feeling that death happens to other people in a remote way can contribute to the feeling of detachment despite the enormity of these events.

Computer games, played by children and young people, regularly contain the opportunity to 'kill' or 'be killed' as part of the story. Characters, once killed, can often be brought to life again by replaying the game, giving the impression that death is a temporary state.

In popular culture, death is represented in television and films. The death of the character Hayley Cropper in 2013 in the TV soap opera, *Coronation Street* appeared to open up conversations about suicide in terminal illness in a way not seen before. Other television shows have regularly represented death in a variety of ways but rarely has it been seen as peaceful, natural and expected – this would not be a very dynamic storyline. In real life, however, a peaceful, pain-free death is what most of us would want for ourselves and what we try to achieve for the dying people we care for.

Is there a 'right' time to die?

Sometimes, a person approaching the end of their life or their families may ask for an indication of how much time they have left. It is extremely difficult, sometimes impossible, to predict how much time the person has left to live but doctors often use the '**surprise question**', that is, they ask themselves, 'Would you be surprised if this person died in the next 12 months?' If the answer is no, then ideally we want to start working with the person and his family to understand how we can support them. Because we all have different views about what we would want to happen towards the end of our lives, it is important that someone feels able to broach the subject.

The way we think and feel about dying will directly affect the care we deliver. If, for example, you feel that death is always a negative experience, then you might find it challenging to talk with someone who is approaching their own death and feeling positive about it. What death means to us is shaped by many things, some of which we are not always aware of.

In the UK, the average life expectancy is 79.5 for men and 82.5 for women. Because good healthcare from conception onwards is now the norm, we have an expectation that most people who die will do so because of their age or because of diseases such as cancer. There can be the expectation that families will first lose grandparents, then parents. Then the next generation become the older family members, and this seems to be the natural order of family loss. If someone dies before reaching older age, the natural order is disturbed and the death can seem more difficult to accept because of this.

Sometimes people's views of life expectancy are shaped by previous experience, for example. Have you heard people say: 'We [our family] are a long line of survivors, my gran reached 90, her mother reached 95, my Aunty is 85 …'. The unspoken expectation is that everyone will have that experience.

Learning how to react to death

Our first encounter with death and how those around us behave will influence our future thinking. For many people the first experience of death is through the death of family pets.

> Think about the first time a pet died. Was there any acknowledgement of the sadness you felt or was it dismissed as 'just' a pet? Were you able to be involved in disposing of the body? Was the body shown respect?

Your own approach to death

The way we think about death will directly affect the decisions we make and therefore the care that we give. For example, an elderly lady died peacefully and expectedly at home. Her two regular carers arrived shortly after she died and found her lying in her bed, her eyes shut and her large family around her. Her small grandchildren were playing on the floor close to her bed. The two carers had two very different views. For one carer, this was a very natural family scene, the other carer thought it highly inappropriate for children to remain in the same room. One saw a family with someone who had died, the other saw children in the same room as a dead body. Neither view is right or wrong but this example sums up how our view of death will affect the way we care for and respond to people at the end of their life.

When you are working with a team of professional carers or with families, it is important that if they feel they want to talk about dying,

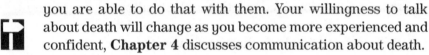 you are able to do that with them. Your willingness to talk about death will change as you become more experienced and confident, **Chapter 4** discusses communication about death.

You need to be aware that many people never wish to talk about death and dying and it is wrong to force them to do so. You need to be willing to talk if they raise the subject but should also be sensitive to the distress which may be caused by starting conversations inappropriately.

On a scale of 1 (not comfortable at all) to 10 (completely comfortable), how comfortable are you discussing death? Have you ever discussed their death with your older relatives? Do you think you know enough to be able to be able to say what they want at the end of their lives?

Have you thought about your own death? What would you want to happen?

If you ask family and friends what kind of death they would want for themselves, you will probably find a mix between those who want to die quickly so they are not aware, and those who want to have time to prepare, put their personal and legal business in order. Throughout the chapters in this book, you will be given the opportunity to reflect on different aspects of dying.

Try to think about your own thoughts and feelings as well as the people you are caring for.

Thinking about dying: things to remember

The work of looking after dying people and their families can be very emotional, particularly if you know them well or the circumstances are difficult. Providing professional compassionate care can be challenging as there is a balance between forming a personal connection, which allows you to show empathy, and maintaining the distance which allows you to behave appropriately as their caregiver.

Being aware of how you are feeling about the situations you are dealing with, and how your behaviour and actions are affecting others, will help you to achieve that balance. Caring for people at the end of their life can be draining, both physically and emotionally. In **Chapter 11** you will find examples of how you can look after yourself.

What does end of life mean?

Liz Reed

Facing the end of life can be very frightening. But what does it really mean? Does it mean years, months, weeks, days? In reality, it can mean different things to different people.

This chapter will consider:

- what we mean by end of life;
- the different terms you might hear and useful definitions of end of life and palliative care;
- what the course of different illnesses might look like;
- advance care planning;
- decision-making and issues around Do Not Attempt Cardiopulmonary Resuscitation (DNACR) orders;
- predicting and preparing for the final stages of life.

Some people will live for years after the diagnosis of a life-limiting illness, knowing that they cannot be cured, while others deteriorate rapidly, giving them little time to think about the end of their life and how they would wish their care to be. The course of illness can be complicated. Sometimes there may be many options for treatment which means people can be very unwell, receive treatment to control the effects of the illness and temporarily feel better. These cycles of treatment and improved moments of health can go on for years, making it very difficult to predict when the end of life is going to come, as it may have been anticipated many times. What we do know is that different illness at the end of life may follow a particular pattern. We will explore these patterns and the challenges of predicting the **end stage** for people in this chapter.

Making decisions and planning for the end of life can be upsetting and hard for people to think and talk about, particularly when they are trying to focus on feeling better. We will look at how we can support people to have these conversations and document their wishes. **Advance care planning (ACP)** will be discussed, how to go about this, the challenges of carrying it out, and how you may be able to support people through the processes of planning for the end of life.

What are some of the words you have heard in relation to end of life care, for example, palliative care and terminal care? What do you think they mean?

Words associated with dying

Talking about the end of life with people can be difficult when we all use different words to describe it: **palliative care**, **terminal care**, **life-threatening**, **life-limiting**, **incurable** and **hospice care**. To people unfamiliar with them, these terms can be confusing and they may feel as though they give mixed messages.

Below are the definitions of palliative and end of life care. What do you notice when you look at the two definitions? Are there similarities or differences? What do you think are the important messages in both definitions that support good care? How do they compare with your definitions and the care that you provide?

Palliative care: an approach that improves the quality of life of people with life-threatening illness and their families facing the problem associated with life-threatening illness, through the pre-vention and relief of suffering by means of early identification and impeccable assessment and treatment of pain and other problems, physical, psychosocial and spiritual.

(WHO)

End of life care: helps all those with advanced, progressive, incurable illness to live as well as possible until they die. It enables the supportive and palliative care needs of both patient and family to be identified and met throughout the last phase of life and into bereavement. It includes management of pain and other symptoms and provision of psychological, social, spiritual and practical support.

(Department of Health 2008)

To complicate things, the term palliative care is often associated with dying, even though the definition states that it aims to help people to live well before they die. In reality, the definitions are alike and not just associated with the very last days or weeks of life. End of life care begins when needed, and continues for as long as it is needed. According to the General Medical Council (GMC) definition, patients are approaching the end of life when they are assessed by those responsible for their care as likely to die within the next 12 months – this includes patients living with advanced incurable conditions which may cause them to die in the next few weeks or months or years.

So we can describe **end of life care**, but is this the same as the end stage?

When is the end stage?

The **end stage** is difficult to predict as no two people are the same and there are many different types of illnesses which follow different paths or patterns. Some people will consider they are at the end of their life when they find out they have an incurable illness even though they may live for months or years. Other people will consider they are at the end of their life when they have deteriorated and feel dependent on others. They may have a very short time to live. End of life care usually means the period of time before the person dies a natural death (a death by natural causes usually as a result of illness as opposed to unnatural death, for example, suicide, murder or accident). This is often considered to be the last 6 or 12 months of life, while the end of life phase (often also called the terminal phase) is usually considered to be the last month, weeks or days before the person dies. This is often a time when the person and those around them recognise that they are changing, deteriorating or worsening without the possibility of improvement. The deaths we are talking about in the book are natural deaths.

Can you predict when someone is entering the end of their life?

Doctors and nurses are often asked by people with serious advanced illness: 'How long have I got?' Healthcare staff are usually reluctant to give specific answers and often will use phrases such as 'Short weeks' or 'A few short months.' This is because it can be very difficult to predict. No two people will follow exactly the same pattern of deterioration towards the end of life, even with the same illness. Below are examples of different illnesses and the pattern they may follow with the progression of the illness. The pattern of change in the way illness affects a person is sometimes called an **illness trajectory**.

Three different trajectories of dying help us to understand the patterns of deterioration we might see:

1. The first trajectory is represented by short period of illness with a fairly predictable deterioration in health over weeks, months or years. People with cancer are more likely to follow this trajectory. During this time they may have a period of wellness as a result of treatment. Over time, their physical ability will deteriorate and they commonly experience **fatigue,** weight loss, pain and other symptoms. The final decline is likely to be a slow deterioration in their mobility and ability to care for themselves. This decline may continue steadily until death.
2. The second trajectory is commonly seen in long-term conditions, such as chronic heart failure and chronic obstructive pulmonary disease. It is characterised by a slow deterioration, often over years, with acute events such as chest infections or shortness of breath which may need treatment, requiring care at home or hospital admission. While people can survive these events, it is likely that their health and ability to care for themselves will deteriorate over time. The symptoms of those with chronic heart failure and chronic obstructive pulmonary disease are often managed with a number of different treatments but as time goes by, the treatment becomes less effective. A decline in the person's ability to look after themselves and an increasing number of acute events with little apparent benefit from a change in treatment may indicate that they are closer to the end of their lives.
3. The third trajectory has been described as 'prolonged dwindling' (Murray et al. 2005). People experiencing this are more likely to be elderly, frail and experiencing illness associated with older

age such as dementia and multiple health problems. These people will experience a gradual deterioration in physical and mental ability. For others, the ageing process is a gradual decline in both physical ability and memory, meaning they need help with all aspects of their daily living. The end of life can be associated with an acute event such as a fall or chest infection (Lunney et al. 2003; Murray et al. 2005).

These three trajectories show how difficult it can be to plan for the end of life as it is difficult to predict what will happen and when. This can make it challenging to think when the best time to talk about end of life care is.

When do we talk about end of life?

Have you ever talked to your family about what you (or they) would want to happen at the end of your life?

- What care you would like at the end of your life?
- Who would you like to be there?
- Where would you like to be?
- What treatment would you consider acceptable?
- What do you think you would refuse?
- Would you plan the funeral?
- How would it feel to have these conversations?
- What may stop you?

Many people are uncomfortable talking about the end of life. It can be a difficult thing to face and many people prefer to avoid the topic rather than upsetting the people that they care about. This can make it challenging to know when is the best time to talk about end of life care.

In order to ensure that we are providing the care people want, where possible, people need to be involved in decisions about their care and who provides it. We cannot know what people want unless we ask them. The earlier in their illness that people can consider it, the better planned they can be for the remainder of their life. This is particularly important if the person has an illness which will reduce their ability to be involved in decisions about their care as the illness progresses, for example, dementia. This can be very hard to think about if they have just been given a diagnosis and they know the treatment is not going to cure them.

For some people, when they know they have an illness that will end their life, they are able to talk about and plan for it. Others may not feel able to acknowledge the end of life is close, even when they are very weak and unwell. Some people will never be able to think or talk about the fact that they are at the end of life even when it is obvious to everyone else around them.

So there is no real right or wrong time for people to talk about their wishes at the end of life but, in general, it is good to take time to plan ahead when people are able. The important thing is for them to have the opportunity to talk about this with people they trust and time to consider the end of their life and what they may want.

While we know generally what to expect for different illnesses, the reality is that every person you care about is an individual with a past and a future unique to them. This should be at the front of your mind when considering the needs of each person you care about; it should be tailored to their specific needs. This is often referred to as 'personalised care'. Personalisation of care means that whoever receives support, whether this comes from health or social care services or they fund it themselves, is entitled to be involved in decisions about the care they receive, the quality of that care, and control over how this is provided. To find out more about communication skills and how to have difficult conversations, look at **Chapter 4**.

Making decisions about end of life care: what do people really want?

Making decisions about whether to accept treatment or not can be very hard for a person when they know the treatment will not cure them. People can feel pressure from those around them to accept treatment which may extend their life but to them it may also mean disruption, discomfort and unpleasant side-effects which affect their quality of life. Sometimes people say 'no' to treatment which may only give them temporary relief. This can be harder than saying 'yes' to treatment. Such conversations can lead to division within families. Some people will choose quality of life over quantity of life, and while it is important that you don't influence their decision, allowing them to talk about their options and listening to what is important may help them feel clearer about what they want to do.

Some people choose not to be involved in discussions about their treatment and care but they may have views on where they would prefer to be cared for, who they would like to be cared for by, who they would want with them and where they would wish to be when they die. While some people may want to talk to their doctor about this, it is possible that they will choose someone with whom they have developed a relationship with and whom they trust. You may be the person they choose to talk to, so it is important for you to consider how you would handle this situation.

Maria's story

This is part of Maria's story. She is one of three people we are following throughout this book.

Think about how you would cope if you were in the following situation and someone was talking to you about their approaching death.

You are very busy and there are not enough staff and too many things to do. You are helping wash Maria when, out of the blue, she says, 'I don't think I'm going to live much longer and I always wanted to die here at home.' What would you do?

1. *Tell her not to be silly, she's doing fine?*
2. *Explore why she thinks this?*
3. *Discuss what her wishes for end of life care are?*
4. *Focus on what you are doing and say nothing?*

On a busy day with so much to do, the easy option may be to say nothing or dismiss Maria's concerns. Time is something you don't have. But this may be the only time she has felt able to express her wishes and if you don't acknowledge them, she may not achieve them. People often talk about concerns when they are relaxed and doing something familiar. Think about what you should do and how you would go about it. Remember that you are also working as a member of a larger team with other professions. A **multiprofessional team** approach is important in supporting your care of Maria.

To explore these difficult subjects you should think about a number of things:

- *Location*: ideally, to talk these things through, you will need to be somewhere quiet and private where you won't be disturbed and Maria can feel safe. You may have to politely ask other people to leave.
- *Goals*: what is important for her – you may suspect she is approaching the end of life but does she hope for more treatment? Her goals may be very simple or very complicated but should be the centre of any discussion.
- *Time*: make sure you have plenty of time and that you will not need to rush off to do something else. If you are unable to talk at the time, you should tell her that you would like to come back when you know you will have more time.
- *Support*: who would Maria like to have with her when considering these issues? For example, she may want to include a friend or her family in the discussions.
- *Action*: what action can you take to enable Maria to achieve her preferred place of care and place of death?
- *Barriers*: what barriers are there which may prevent Maria achieving her preferred place of care and place of death?
- *Documentation*: what documentation will you need to ensure you record the decisions about her preferred place of care and preferred place of death where others involved in the care can access it? This includes the home, hospital or a care home, to ensure all those involved in her care are aware of any documented preferences and can easily access the information.
- *Communication*: open, clear, sensitive communication is important for Maria to express what is important to her.

How would you communicate all decisions and plans with Maria and those around her to ensure she is involved in the whole process?

 Look at **Chapter 4**.

The process of helping people plan their future is referred to as advance care planning (ACP). This plan is designed to help people live and die in the place of their choice and to have some control over the care they receive. Helping someone to achieve their wishes at the end of life can be really rewarding despite the challenges.

Given the choice, most people choose to die in their own homes. Not many would choose to die in a hospital yet the majority of people do. For many, they have never been given the chance to think about and decide where they would like to be cared for and where they want to be when they die. So it is important that those involved in the care of the person who is going to die give them the opportunity to talk about it and decide. Even though these conversations are difficult, they need to happen. Even if the person doesn't want to talk about it, introducing the idea means they may come back to it at a later date.

What do we mean by advance care planning?

We have already talked about how important it is for people to be able to plan ahead, particularly if they are going to be unable to make decisions as their illness progresses. ACP is a structured process of discussing with people and their families their wishes for care towards the end of their lives and documenting this.

Advance care planning ensures people can express their wishes about the following:

- where they want to be cared for at the end of their life;
- what care and treatment they want at the end of their life;
- what they don't want to happen at the end of their life;
- who will act for them if they are unable to act for themselves.

ACP allows people to contribute to decisions about a time in their future care when they may lose the ability to make decisions as a result of illnesses, such as dementia or other changes in their condition, and they may wish to appoint someone they trust to ensure their wishes are honoured by registering someone with **lasting power of attorney (LPA)**. Some care homes have advance care plans as part of their assessment on admission. We know that those with an advance care plan are more likely to have the care at the end of life that they want to have but they may also help family members to consider their role both in the present and the future and ultimately may help in their bereavement if the end of life was as their relative wanted.

It is important to remember that advance care plans should be kept up to date and reviewed regularly. People sometimes change their minds, their circumstances may change or they may see the situation in a different way. It is important that any changes are reported and recorded in the official documentation so that any change in what the person wants can be met.

DNACPR (Do Not Attempt Cardiopulmonary Resuscitation) may be a phrase you have heard. ACP allows people the opportunity to state their preferences for resuscitation and in what circumstances it should be applied. It can be challenging to consider planning end of life care, so good communication and shared decision-making between the healthcare staff and the person dying are very important. The dying person needs those responsible for their care to give them all the accurate information they need to make an informed decision and the doctors and other healthcare staff must listen to what the person wants and support their decision. DNACPR decisions do need to be considered in end of life care. They apply only to cardiopulmonary resuscitation (CPR). CPR is the act of restarting the heart (and lungs) when they have stopped. CPR can be difficult for healthcare professionals and patients and their families to consider. DNACPR does not withhold other treatments or care. People can confuse these things and worry that those with a DNACPR decision will have nutrition and fluid withdrawn, which is not true.

Main points when considering DNACPR:

- Consider it as part of advance care planning with a person.
- Ensure the dying person understands what it is and what it isn't.
- Reassure the person that DNACPR decisions can be changed.
- The decision made should be reviewed frequently considering both the illness and the wishes of the person which may change.
- It is different from ACP but may be part of it.
- DNACPR decisions apply only to resuscitate if the heart stops – not to any other interventions such as infection requiring antibiotics.

Those responsible for the person's care should ensure that a DNACPR form is clearly written and available for everyone involved in the care. That means it should be copied to everyone involved in the care and visible in the person's home. If there is no documented DNACPR and an ambulance is called to a patient who has collapsed, they are duty-bound to resuscitate that person and take them to the nearest Accident and Emergency Department. This can be highly distressing for both the dying person and the family if they had agreed a DNACPR previously.

Albert's preferences

Shortly after Albert moved to Holly House Care Home, it was suggested that his preferences for future care should be discussed. Albert made an advance care plan with his niece, Jackie, and those responsible for his care, but it was difficult because he was weak and had difficulty expressing what he wanted. But he was clear that he wanted to stay where he was. He has always said that, when the time came, he didn't want anyone to 'jump on his chest'. When his niece asked him about this, despite his frailty, he was adamant that he did not want to be resuscitated in the event of his heart or breathing stopping. He was reassured that everything would be done to ensure his wishes were respected. The doctor documented Albert's DNACPR decision and made sure the care home staff were aware. It was also agreed that Jackie should have lasting power of attorney. He has always trusted his only niece.

Think about when the best time to prepare an ACP might be. At diagnosis, or perhaps when the person is deteriorating? How would you go about ensuring your patient has the option to plan for their future place of care and place of death? What would you do with that information?

The decision-making process should include all those involved in the care, including the family, to develop a final document which includes the person's wishes. As someone involved in the care of people who will die, it is important that you consider advance care planning with others responsible for their care, such as doctors, nurses, social workers and care workers. These sort of things should be discussed as part of multiprofessional meetings which include, where possible, the person and their family members.

Talking to people and their relatives about planning end of life care

Talking about their end of life care and dying can be hard and, at times, overwhelming for the person who knows they will die and equally for their family and friends. As someone looking after a person who is dying, you too may worry that you won't be able to cope with the emotions it brings up. No-one wants to cause others distress or see them upset so you may think it is easier not to have those difficult conversations. However hard, giving the person the time and opportunity to talk about what the future holds and what they see as their future care will help both of you understand what their wishes are. Being able to tell someone what their fears are and the care they want can be a huge relief.

Not everyone will be able to consider the end of their life, even if to you it seems close. So it is important to take your lead from the person. To do this, you will need to gently and sensitively explore whether the person has considered what their wishes would be towards the end of their life. Again, this includes what treatment would be acceptable and whether they have thought about where they would like to be cared for towards the end of their life. Even if someone chooses not to talk about care towards the end of their life, don't assume they never will. Tell them they can talk about it at a later time. Give the person time to reflect on advance care planning. It may be that they wish to talk to a member of their family or take time to consider what they really want towards the end of their life. National Health Service (NHS) guidance on ACP states that advance care plans should be:

- documented;
- regularly reviewed;
- communicated to key persons involved in their care;
- if the individual wishes, their family and friends may be included.

(Department of Health 2008)

There is no official document that everyone uses to record an advance care plan but there should be a policy recognised as the correct way in your organisation. It should include a document which is accessible to the person who is dying, their family and everyone else involved in their care.

What are the challenges to advance care planning?

As we have already discussed, some people will never want to plan their care in advance. Before introducing the idea of ACP, think of any issues that may be significant, for example, the person's background, community, beliefs and values. Some people may not be comfortable with planning for the end of life. See **Chapter 8**.

These difficult discussions can bring up strong emotions in all involved which is entirely normal. Done well, advance care planning can be a great relief for the person, their family and those responsible for their care.

Family members may not want you to talk about planning for the future. They may put up barriers to avoid such conversations. Try and take time to talk to them about their concerns and why it is helpful to think about what would be important to their relative towards the end of their life. Reassure them that by documenting their wishes, everyone involved in their care will have a copy and do everything possible to ensure they are respected.

If the wishes of the person who is going to die are not communicated and made accessible to everyone involved in their care, the process can fail. Make sure the advance care plan is easily accessible and copies are where people can find them. If in the home, everyone should know where it is. If a paramedic is called, they will need to see the advance care plan, otherwise they are obliged to take the person to the nearest Accident and Emergency Department.

What happens when the person is not able to make decisions for themselves?

While the family of those with life-limiting illness may influence their care or act in their best interests, in order to ensure the care their relative wanted at the end of their life, they may need to consider taking on a lasting power of attorney. A lasting power of attorney permits the person to appoint others to make decisions on their behalf. This is a legally binding document for people who see a time ahead when they may be unable to manage their personal and legal affairs and health and welfare. The lasting power of attorney documents whoever has been appointed to make decisions on behalf of the ill person and their wishes in advance of a time when they no longer have capacity to act for themselves.

There are two types of lasting power of attorney:

- health and welfare;
- property and financial affairs.

Health and welfare lasting power of attorney

If the person is unable to make their own decisions, they identify one or more people to make decisions about things like:

- daily living activities (such as eating, washing and dressing);
- medical care;
- whether an alternative place of care would be in their best interests;
- treatment, including interventions that may maintain life.

Property and financial affairs lasting power of attorney

The person appointed to be the lasting power of attorney is able to act on behalf of the person who is dying to:

- pay bills;
- collect benefits;
- sell property.

If anyone in your care has a lasting power of attorney, you should ensure it is well documented and all those involved in their care are aware of it. A lasting power of attorney is prepared by a solicitor working on the person's behalf.

Preparing for the end of life

For many, preparing for the end of life is an important way to ease the burden on family and friends. People may talk of 'getting their affairs in order', which can mean their financial affairs as well as considering other matters that will be dealt with after they have gone, such as funeral arrangements, last will and testament or memories and mementoes to be left for family or friends. Doing all these things can help to ease the worry of leaving loved ones behind. As someone caring for them, they may want you to help them with preparations so having an understanding of these things can be helpful. If the person has no last will and testament, they will need to speak to a solicitor to arrange the details of what their wishes are.

Take time to give people the opportunity to discuss what they might want at the end of life and beyond for those they leave behind. Some people will never be able to plan ahead for themselves or those around them, as someone responsible for their care; you will have to accept that different people adjust and cope in different ways and not force anyone to face something they cannot. Your role may then turn to supporting those they leave behind.

What does end of life mean? Things to remember

- Supporting and caring for people towards the end of their life, allowing them the space to talk about their fears and tell you what their wishes are and doing all you can to ensure their wishes are respected are the essence of good end of life care.
- It is important to remember that end of life means different things to different people.
- Decisions regarding end of life care sometimes need to be made and advance care planning discussed and communicated.

The nature of a person's illness can be a predictor of the end stages of their life. Now we have considered how we support people to plan for the end of live and the ways of doing this, **Chapter 3** will consider where they may choose to be cared for at the at the end of life. It will also consider the different care professional and agencies that may be involved in this care.

Where are people cared for and who is involved?

Karen Cook and Beverly Clayton

Care for those approaching the end of their lives takes place in many different settings: hospitals, hospices, care homes or the person's own home. This chapter will consider:

- the importance of recognising those individuals with end of life care needs requiring ongoing support over months or years;
- how to recognise those individuals with end of life care needs whose condition is rapidly deteriorating and where they may die in weeks, days or hours;
- care provision in a person's own home or in a care home; and the impact place of care has on the support they may require;
- who may be involved in the care and support of a person with end of life care needs.

An estimated half a million people die in the United Kingdom (about 1 per cent of the population) each year. When asked, only 8 per cent of the population said that they would choose to die in hospital, with the vast majority, over two-thirds, stating that they would choose to die where they live. Despite this, of those people who die in the UK each year, around a staggering 58 per cent die in hospital (Department of Health 2008). In some cases this will be out of choice because their situation has become difficult to maintain because of the changes in their condition and/or because of the level of support that is possible. Many people will not achieve their preferred place of care or indeed preferred place of death.

This situation is slowly changing with the knowledge of how important it is to ask people about these preferences, to record and share these and then plan care to support the achievement of their preference. This chapter will illustrate some of the ways people may be supported to achieve their choices.

People at the end of their life may be supported by many different people from social care or healthcare services, by families and friends or voluntary services. The type of support available will be in response to the individual needs of the person requiring assistance and care. The care provided will depend on their general condition and whether this is changing due to their ill health. Support may come from those already involved in care or require the involvement of different care professionals or specialist services; often these professionals would take on the role of the individual's key worker. These various roles and services will also be considered in this chapter.

The place of care will be considered and comparisons made between the care of the person in their own home and those in residential care settings. While similar principles apply to those being cared for in a hospital or hospice, this will not be considered here as supporting people to remain in their usual place of care is the priority for the majority of people and services. The main focus will centre on the two groups of people who may be cared for as the end of life approaches:

- those requiring on-going support over months or years;
- those whose condition is rapidly deteriorating where their death may be in weeks, days or hours.

Those requiring care and support over months or years

When you think about a person who may be entering the last part of their lives, what changes might you notice in their appearance, behaviour and activity? And how do you think these changes could affect the care and support they require?

When an individual is recognised as entering the last part of their life, it may be necessary to review the support they require. This should be done through discussion with the person affected and those close to them, giving everyone an opportunity to outline their wishes and preferences for their future care. It requires sensitive conversations and some understanding by the individual that their circumstances and health have changed. This crucial conversation can help us to provide **person-centred care** by discovering what is important to the individual – information that can then be recorded and shared, with the person's permission, with those who are involved in supporting them. This process of open and honest discussion, recording and sharing information is called **advance care planning** (ACP) and has been discussed in **Chapter 2**.

Assessing the individual and discovering whether any changes are taking place is vital in helping to recognise their changing needs and supporting these. When a person's condition is deteriorating or changing and they need additional support, you may see some or all of the changes below. It is important to discover whether these are new problems or the worsening of existing issues:

- They may require more assistance with basic functions, e.g. preparing food, shopping, cleaning, clothes washing.
- They may struggle to have a wash or get dressed.
- They may find moving around more challenging.
- They may complain that their appetite is small or that they have little interest in food.
- They may feel more tired, even when they are resting or napping.
- They may feel less inclined to socialise with their family and friends.
- They may complain of new or worsening symptoms (see **Chapter 5**).

Types of care provided

In the UK, there are different ways of providing care. This could be achieved through social care services. These services help people who are in need of support due to illness, disability or old age. Services can also support the families or carers of people receiving social care. Services could include, for example, personal help around the house, changes to help the person move around their house, or even an alarm system so that they can call for help if needed. Often the care provided is described as a 'package of care'. Social care is subject to rules about the person's needs and ability. Local authorities (councils) are responsible for providing social care services for those who need them and are eligible for them. To enable this care to be supported, the person would be reviewed by a member of the local social care team. These care services are often 'means tested' – this means that the person's financial situation, savings and income are also reviewed alongside their needs. After these assessments, the local authority may agree to pay either in full or partially for the care and support needed. Social care services may be provided by 'independent providers' – firms or charities who specialise in providing social care services. Social care services can take many forms and you can get help from them while you live at home, out and about in the community, or even in a new place of residence such as a care home. In the community, in the person's home, this could include help with personal care such as helping a person to wash and dress, go to the toilet, prepare and eat simple meals, help with cleaning and shopping.

Another way of providing care is through **NHS continuing healthcare**. NHS continuing healthcare is free care outside of hospital that is arranged and funded by the NHS. It is only available for people who need ongoing healthcare and meet the eligibility criteria. To be eligible for NHS continuing healthcare, the person must be assessed as having a **'primary health need'** and have a complex medical condition and substantial and ongoing care needs. NHS continuing healthcare can be provided in any setting, including a care home, some hospices or the home of the person. If someone in a care home is receiving NHS continuing healthcare, it will cover their care home fees, including the cost of accommodation, personal care and healthcare costs. If NHS continuing healthcare is provided in the home of the person, it will cover personal care and healthcare costs. To access this way of providing care requires referral and assessment by the continuing healthcare team, a process that is supported by additional information available from those healthcare professionals involved in the person's care.

The provision of care, the benefits and welfare system are complex and ever changing. For up-to-date information about the different ways of accessing care, go to the NHS Choices website (www.nhs. uk). There are also different benefits that may be available to the person and their main carer, to find out more about benefits in the UK, go to the UK government's website (www.gov.uk). Another source of information and advice is the Citizens Advice Bureau: they provide free, independent, confidential and impartial advice to everyone on their rights and responsibilities. The **Appendix** provides a list of helpful web addresses.

Find out how to refer to the local social care team. Find out how to refer to the continuing healthcare team in your local area. Find out the referral criteria for both services.

Care for a person in their own home

Albert has dementia

Albert has dementia. He often forgets to eat and worryingly leaves food in the fridge for days until it is inedible. He has 'mates' and his niece Jackie. Jackie visits as often as she can, but has her own young family. For most of the time, Albert is home alone. The house is dishevelled and so is Albert. He often forgets to dress or wash or even drink. He can get quite angry and irritable if Jackie mentions that things seem to be getting on top of him. Albert seems to be sleeping for long periods of the day and often takes an age to come to the door when his friends visit.

What help do you think Albert might need? Can you think of any challenges in setting this up for Albert?

When caring for someone in their own home, there are some important questions to ask:

- How is the person coping? And also those close to them?
- Do they live alone?
- Are they cared for by their partner? Is their carer elderly or do they have their own health problems?
- Is it a daughter or son looking after an elderly parent? Do they have young children or other caring responsibilities?
- Is the environment appropriate? Is more equipment or adaptation required or does furniture need to be moved?

Some of these questions will be answered by direct questioning but others may be through observation, such as the number of family members, friends and neighbours involved in supporting the person and the frequency and level of support provided, i.e. if the person cannot be left alone, if the family are helping them to eat or to wash.

A carer assessment can be requested and would be carried out by the social care team. This can help support the carer by providing either vouchers or a direct payment to support respite care – this could be through the provision of a paid carer in the home, or in a care facility, i.e. a care home. Respite offers care for the individual so that the family or friends can have a short break from caring. This break could be a few hours on a regular basis at home so that the family member can leave the person in safe hands; or a longer period of care, for example, in a care home with nursing. Often this can mean the difference between the person and their loved ones coping or struggling.

Find out how to refer to the social care team for a carer assessment.

As well as statutory services (i.e. those supported by social services or healthcare), there may be additional services available in your area to support people in their own homes. One example is 'Crossroads', a national organisation that supports those engaged in care giving by offering respite at home for the individual they are responsible for. During this period the individual is supported in their own home for a few hours at a time by a trained care support worker, enabling the family member to carry out tasks which they need to do and may not be able to do when they are with their loved one, or have a break and leave the home to meet friends, for example. In some places this may incur a cost.

Some areas may also have voluntary services. Volunteers will stay with an individual in their own home while their family member or carer leaves the house for a short period.

Find out about the different services available in your local area. Why not try your local council's website? Here you may find contacts for local organisations and groups.

Albert's move to a care home

Following a case conference between Albert, his niece Jackie, his GP and his social worker, it was decided that he should move to a care home. She was finding it increasingly difficult to care for him and his dementia meant that he was becoming increasingly aggressive when anyone went to the house to help. His social worker offered to take him to look at two homes that had space for him but he said he did not care just as long as he did not have to share a room. Holly House, a care home with nursing and a wing dedicated to the care of people with dementia was selected and he moved in willingly and seemed relieved that he would no longer have to cope on his own. Because of his health needs, his place at the home was fully funded and only 30 minutes drive from Jackie and her family which suited them both.

Care in a care home

Just under half a million people live in care homes (Department of Health 2008); that's about 1 per cent of the population. According to Age UK (2014), there is an increase in the number of people being cared for in care homes. This rise may be due in part to the increasingly ageing population but also because in society there are less 'nuclear' families with adult children living away from their parents and so unable to actively get involved in their care; adult children may have the pressure of work and their other family commitments.

Care homes can be broadly divided into two types: those that employ registered nurses and so can provide care with nursing; and those that provide support through care support staff. People resident in care homes with nursing (nursing homes) often require a higher level of care input usually because their health and general condition require greater assistance and the skills of trained nurses. For those who live in a care home without nursing (a residential care home), residents are often frail but more able to support some of their own care needs with a little help from the trained care staff. Because of the different ways these homes are staffed and the different ways care is supported, there may also be different people, professionals and services available to both.

As with caring for people in their own homes, it is important that through conversation and observation we discover what is normal for the person. We need to think about how an individual's needs may have changed and if these needs have been slowly changing over some time. It may be noticeable that the person requires more support and that this now needs the assistance of more than one member of staff. Carers may be struggling to help move someone from their bedroom to the sitting room or even a short distance to the bathroom. Use the list later in this chapter to identify if there are general changes in the individual's condition.

In residential care (or care homes without nursing), this may mean that the person requires review either by a social care team or by a healthcare professional to determine if there is an increase in their needs. In care homes with nursing, it may help identify the need for additional time and help staff to provide appropriate care. Here are some of those people who may be available to support and provide help:

- *Core community staff* – General practitioner (GP). If the person is being cared for in their usual place of residence, their GP will remain responsible for their care. The core community staff also includes the district nursing team (own home and residential care), and the community matron.
- *Specialist community staff* – Community speech and language therapist, community **occupational therapist**, community physiotherapist, community dietician, domiciliary opticians, dentists, chiropodists.
- *Condition-specific staff* – Heart failure nurse specialist, respiratory care team, multiple sclerosis nurse specialist, Motor Neuron Disease Association, tissue viability nurse, community psychiatric nurse, Admiral nurse (dementia) or dementia navigator, cancer nurse specialist, Macmillan nurse, palliative care nurse specialist.

This list is not exhaustive and there will be geographical differences. There will be other services in your area that are available that you wish to add. Even the person with the most straightforward needs can come into contact with many different professionals. Each has a distinct role to play in the person's care and these are outlined at the end of this chapter. It is, however, worth remembering how potentially confusing this can be for a person and their family. Sometimes what they most need is someone to help them to 'navigate' their way through.

Think about where you work; find out which of these roles are available to help support residents in your care and how you can contact them.

So far in this chapter, we have considered the different needs someone may have depending on where they are cared for. It is also important to consider that there may be differences in their life expectancies. Some people will survive for months or years but their last few days or weeks sees a rapid change in their condition. Others may enter this phase or rapid deterioration much more quickly. The chapter will continue by looking at those who are in a state of rapid decline.

Those requiring care and support when their condition is rapidly deteriorating

We have considered the changes that occur in someone's condition, changes that help identify that a person may be entering the last months or years of their lives. Now think about what other changes you might notice if they are imminently dying in the next few days.

You may notice that the individual is experiencing some or all of these difficulties;

- They may be generally restless, finding it difficult to settle.
- They may be a little muddled or confused.
- They may have become more withdrawn and either unable to or not wanting to socialise.
- They may be more sleepy, fatigued and lethargic.
- They may be taking in less food and fluids.
- They may struggle to catch their breath or become easily out of breath even with little exertion.
- They may say that they are seeing people who have already died.

- They may say that they are dying.
- They may feel that they have 'unfinished business' to settle.
- Their skin integrity may be compromised, leaving them at risk of pressure-related wounds and poor wound healing.
- They may experience swelling in their feet and ankles – this would be a new problem for this person.

This list can be used to assess the person you are caring for. Now ask yourself, have they had similar episodes in the past? In the past had this been a temporary worsening of their condition which then resolved spontaneously or with treatment? For more information about managing symptoms and care in the last few hours of life, refer to **Chapters 5 and 6**.

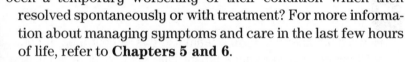

Maria's breathlessness

Maria often experiences episodes of breathlessness. She is aware that the hospital team are unable to offer her any new medications to better manage her heart failure and its associated breathlessness. Most of the time when she is breathless, she coughs up frothy white phlegm (a sign of her heart failure) – this is quite usual for Maria. On this occasion though, she feels very unwell. She struggles to keep awake, she seems a little muddled not sure of the day, time or her location. She turns her daughter Lily away when she comes to visit. She is producing rather grey-green-coloured phlegm and feels very hot to the touch.

What would you be thinking if you were caring for Maria? Do you think there may be something else going on or do you think she is entering the last few days of her life, and what would this mean for her care?

For those individuals who may be suffering a temporary and possibly reversible change in their condition, additional support for care at home may be available from a team working in the community who provide short-term support until the person has returned to their usual functioning. These teams can have different names and there will be local variations – in some areas they are the

'Re-enablement team', they could be the 'Intermediate Care team' or 'Response & Rehab team'. Their involvement can be requested from the GP, Community Matron, district nurse or social services – this may be different depending on where you work. They can support care on a temporary basis for usually no more than 6 weeks after which point they will either withdraw or refer to either social care services or continuing healthcare team for a continued package of care.

Find out whether you have a team like this in your area. If not, find out how you would arrange urgent care support on a temporary or short-term basis in a person's own home.

Do these changes represent a situation which cannot be reversed with treatment or medications? If this is the case, it may be that the person is entering the final few days or weeks of their life. Any decision about this is best made by all those who know and are involved in the person's care – this can include their GP, family, district nurse, care home staff, therapists and any other professional carer who knows the person.

Once recognition of the person's irreversible and deteriorating condition has been agreed, services may vary depending on where they are being cared for.

Supporting care of the person in their own home

Many people are cared for in their own home, often with their primary carer being their partner or immediate family. The principles of care are similar to those previously discussed; however, the GP is more actively involved as the end of life approaches, with the support of other care professionals as needed.

GP practices have certain services supporting their surgery. An important one is the district nursing team. This team is able to support the individual by offering nursing care in the person's own home and works closely with the GP. Nursing care may include, for example; continence assessment, such as the need for pads or a urinary catheter; wound care; assessment of the person's pressure areas; administration of medications. There may also be a community matron involved with the person's care particularly if they have long-term chronic medical conditions, if so, has the community matron been involved with the assessment? If not, ask their opinion.

Maria's deterioration

Maria was aware of her failing health. Her GP liaised with the hospital cardiology team and heart failure nurse to check that there was no possibility of additional treatment and that her current deteriorating condition could not be reversed. The GP informed Maria and Aldo of the situation, a situation that they both had suspected; and discussed this with the other members of the family (at Maria and Aldo's request) and then with the district nurse. They all confirmed that the deterioration in Maria's condition was likely to end in her death and that her choice was to die in her own home. The district nurses visited later that day to introduce themselves and offer their support. Maria and her family declined the offer of extra help with care when the district nurse suggested referring them to the local end of life care rapid response team. Maria's family felt that they could support the more practical aspects of their mum's care.

The person and their family may need help with practical care, i.e. hygiene needs, changing bedding, moving them in their bed, etc. If the person already has care provided, it may be necessary to increase the frequency of visits and the number of care staff required to support the person, i.e. from one carer per visit to two carers per visit. If the care needs to be increased, in this circumstance, the service providing the current care needs to be contacted to support additional care needs.

If the person hasn't required care support at home, there are different teams who may be available in your area to help fill this gap until statutory care is set up. These teams may have different names depending on where you are in the UK. In some areas they are referred to as the Community Hospice and Home Nursing Service and are available via the district nursing service. In other areas they may be described as end of life care rapid response teams. Some will be based in the community alongside district nursing teams, while others may be based at a hospice as part of a hospice at home service.

Find out how to get in touch with district nurses in your area. Find out whether you have an end of life care team available to respond to an individual who is rapidly deteriorating and dying. Keep a note of their contact details and let your team know what support they can offer.

If the person is dying imminently, these teams may be able to continue to support and care for them until their death. If the person's condition, although deteriorating generally, seems to stabilise, this team may 'fast track' an application for more long-term care provided as part of continuing healthcare in the community.

Other services which may be able to offer support at this time include night sitting services, for example, Marie Curie nurses and carers are available in some areas to provide overnight support for the individual and their family. With this and the other end of life care rapid response teams, referral is made via the district nursing team, GP or via the local hospice community services team. **Chapter 9** contains information about what to expect when someone is reaching the last few days and hours of life, and the care that may need to be considered.

Care assessment in a care home

If the person is living in a residential care home, in this circumstance accessing support is similar to that for someone who is being cared for in their own home. Additional support can also be sought from the many different professionals working in the community setting. This can be actioned through the GP, district nurse, community matron or local hospice community services. The GP and/or district nursing team would be your first port of call.

Create a list of contact details for your GP and district nursing team – do you have their usual numbers and their out-of-hours numbers? What about using 111 services if you are not sure?

If the person is living in a nursing home, the GP remains responsible for the person's care. Have you contacted the GP practice to discuss the changes you have recognised in the person's condition? Are there any new symptoms or are the person's symptoms getting worse? If they are new, they will need a GP assessment. If they are a worsening of already present symptoms, what plan was agreed should the symptom re-occur? What has worked for the person in the past? What simple measures might make the person feel more comfortable? For example, do they need a pressure-relieving mattress and **profiling bed**? Do you have medication on hand to give, if necessary, to maintain their comfort? As their condition changes, do you need to consider the number of staff needed to support their individual needs? Can social care or continuing healthcare team support the additional care needs? What simple things can you do to help the person and their family? **Chapter 9** contains information about what to expect when someone is reaching the last few days and hours of life, and the care that may need to be considered.

Some areas may have a specific team of district nurses whose role is to support nursing and residential care home residents, enabling them to remain in their preferred place of care/death in the care home and not be inappropriately admitted to hospital. Find out if there is such a team in your area.

Wherever the person is being cared for, you should work through all of the ways you may be able to help and support the person's changing condition. Some people will have more complex care and symptom needs and so you could consider referral to a **specialist palliative care team** for further advice, support and assessment. These teams may be based at a local hospice as part of their community services or could be an integrated team working both in the hospital and in people's homes.

Find out where your local specialist palliative care team is based. Request information about how they may be able to support the person, their family and your team. Most specialist teams will have written information explaining their role and the services they can

provide. These services may include hands-on care in the community, practical support for staff, education and training, or may serve
in an advisory role. Find out which of these services may be available
in your area and how to make a referral.

Who else is involved in care?

This chapter has looked at the different care and support available when someone is requiring end of life care over months or
years, or when their condition is rapidly changing; if they are in
their own home or being cared for in a nursing or residential care
home. Previously we listed some of the professionals who may be
involved in the person's care; the following illustrations detail the
roles of the many different professionals who may be involved.
Availability of these different professionals may depend on where
you are located. Some will be available in all areas, e.g. GP,
district nurse, while others may be available through social care
teams, community healthcare or specialist services such as hospice teams. Table 3.1 illustrates how complex care services can
be, with lots of different teams, with the GP central to care and
support.

Table 3.1 Who might be involved in supporting end of life care people?

Title or team	Role and information
Physiotherapist	Assess an individual to understand how physical problems may impact on their ability to lead as independent life as they are able; to determine if they can offer support to help reverse any physical issues or assess for the need for adaptation, for instance, through specialist equipment.
	The aim of the interventions is to maintain the person at optimum levels of independence and so enable quality of life.
Occupational therapist	Assesses and analyses functional difficulties within the person's usual daily activities; to determine if they can offer support to help reverse any physical issues or assess for the need for adaptation, for instance, through specialist equipment.
	The aim of the interventions is to maintain patients at optimum levels of independence and so enable quality of life.

Table 3.1 (Continued)

Title or team	Role and information
Speech and language therapist	To provide consultation to patients, families and other care professionals regarding communication, cognition (thinking) and swallowing. To develop strategies to optimise communication and swallowing functioning.
Dietician	To ensure the provision of adequate dietary intake and identification of those who may be at risk of poor nutrition. To assess for reasons causing malnutrition and prevent ensuing complications. To support the person and those close to them through the changes in their nutrition during their illness.
Complementary therapists, e.g. aromatherapist, clinical hypnotherapist, art therapist, massage therapist	Complementary therapies can be a way of communicating care and compassion, nurturing the mind, body and spirit. They are helpful in relieving some of the key symptoms such as anxiety, sleep, breathlessness, fatigue, pain and constipation.
General practitioner (GP)	GPs look after the health of people in their local community and deal with a whole range of health problems. GPs usually work in practices as part of a team, which includes nurses, healthcare assistants, practice managers, receptionists and other staff. Practices also work closely with other healthcare professionals, such as health visitors, specialist nurses, and social services. See NHS Choices (www.nhs.uk)
District nurses	Nursing care can be provided at home rather than in a hospital or nursing home; and this is carried out by community-based district nursing teams. The person you're looking after may need medical or nursing care to help them remain at home. The GP can arrange for NHS services, such as a district or community nurse, to visit to provide nursing care, e.g. give injections, change dressings, etc. The community or district nurse will be able to arrange for a commode, bedpan, and special mattress or incontinence sheets if they are needed. A district nurse can carry out an assessment of the patient's needs and decide, in consultation with the patient and family, what support is required. They also coordinate the patient's care at home. The district nurse works

(Continued)

Table 3.1 (Continued)

Title or team	Role and information
	with other local services to make sure that the right care and support are provided. See NHS Choices (www.nhs.uk)
Community matron	Community matrons provide expert case management for patients with long-term conditions living in a local area with deteriorating health that may result in declining quality of life or potential hospital admission. See Royal College of Nursing (www.rcn.org.uk)
Nurse specialists e.g. Heart failure nurse, Community psychiatric nurse, Tissue viability nurse (wounds and skin care), Admiral nurse or Dementia navigator, Cancer nurse specialist, Macmillan nurse, Motor Neurone Disease nurse, Palliative Care nurse specialist	Specialist nurses are dedicated to a particular area of nursing; caring for patients suffering from long-term conditions and diseases such as cancer, diabetes, Parkinson's, chronic heart failure, dementia, etc. They play a vital role in educating patients on how best to manage their symptoms, as well as offering support following diagnosis. In many cases the involvement of a specialist nurse can prevent patients being re-hospitalised, enabling them to remain in their preferred place of care. See Royal College of Nursing (www.rcn.org.uk)
Hospice and palliative care services	A number of hospice and palliative care teams now provide a hospice at home service, which complements and supplements the service provided by a person's district nurse. Some teams can offer 24-hour nursing care. Community palliative care nurses (often referred to as Macmillan nurses) give specialist advice on managing the symptoms of illness and can also give practical, psychological and emotional support. They are clinical specialists skilled in pain and symptom control. They can be accessed through district nurses or a person's GP. See Macmillan nurses (www.macmillan.org.uk) The hospice at home service or the community specialist nurses may be the way in which hospice services support people at the end of their lives in their usual place of residence. Both are outreach services working from the hospice but out into the community. They come with the support of the many other services which make up a hospice or specialist palliative care team. These can include social workers, counsellors, welfare advisors, physiotherapists and occupational

Table 3.1 (Continued)

Title or team	Role and information
	therapists, complementary therapists, specialist doctors, chaplains – the list is long and may be different depending on the service available in your area.
	Hospices may also have an in-patient unit providing care 24 hours a day. They may also have day care services. Both may be accessed by their outreach teams.
Key worker	A key worker is a healthcare or care professional who, with the patient's consent, takes the lead in coordinating the patient's care. The key worker also acts as the main point of contact for the patient, their carer and all the professionals who are involved in their care.
	See Marie Curie (www.mariecurie.org.uk)

Find out which professionals are available in your area. Where are they based? What are their referral criteria, i.e. what kinds of referrals do they accept? And how do you refer individuals to their teams?

End of life care: things to remember

- It is important to assess and recognise a person who is entering the last few months, weeks, days or hours of their lives.
- Many services are available and all have a part to play in the person's care. It is worth identifying where help can be sought – this may be healthcare or social care but also the voluntary sector.
- People usually know where they want to die, this is usually where they have lived – this *can be* achieved with the right support..

 Chapter 4 will discuss the importance of effective communication skills in end of life care and strategies that may help these discussions.

How can we communicate with people about dying?

Gill Thomas and Amanda Free

This chapter will:

- reflect on the distress that people feel and how to respond;
- explore what good communication is;
- explore how to respond to difficult questions;
- consider the impact on carers;
- encourage you to think about professional boundaries.

Imagine that you are visiting a country where everyone is speaking a language that you do not understand. You have been involved in a road traffic accident. Having arrived in hospital you have become separated from your fellow travellers. You cannot find anyone that speaks your language. You are feeling lost, scared and alone.

This, in a small way, may replicate how frightened and out of control some of the people we look after are feeling at the end of their life. The most important thing that we can do is to listen to someone's story and hope to connect with them. In this chapter we are going to think about what happens to people and their feelings when they are living with the fact that they will soon be dying, and ways in which we can best support and help them through the way we talk and listen to them.

Each person will face the knowledge that they are dying in different ways and will need different levels of support. One thing that almost everyone will want to do, with a few exceptions, is to express what they are thinking about or feeling. This varies dramatically; some people may only ever want to say a few things on a single occasion, others will want to talk through multiple issues on many occasions.

For those who appear not to want to talk at all, we must continue to give them the opportunity, as we can never predict if they may change their mind.

Who may be able to help?

Think what would happen if you suddenly had to face some kind of unexpected crisis in your life or highly distressing news. Who would you want to talk to? Why would you go to them? What is it about the person (or people) that means you would choose them to talk to?

Do you think that you might want to talk to your partner, your parents or other members of your family? What about friends? Would talking to someone who had had the same kind of problem help you? What about talking to someone who might be an expert in the area? Sometimes we might prefer to talk to someone who knows nothing about us, a stranger. These questions help us to understand why someone may choose a specific person to discuss concerns with – this is not necessarily dependent on their role or professional background.

Often people close to you are the first people you want to talk to, but for some people at the end of their life, they would choose someone outside their family whose role is to support people, such as a carer, nurse, counsellor, pastoral care worker or social worker. Think about who could be involved in supporting someone at the end of their life or what service would be involved.

Why it is important for people to talk and feel listened to

Being able to listen and really hear someone's worries and concerns can make a big difference. This can be a difficult thing to do because we often feel the need to do something. Most of us want to fix things and make people feel OK. Someone facing the end of their life is not something that can be easily 'fixed', nor should it be thought about in that way. Sometimes we need to accept that we do not need to know all the answers; it's OK not to know how to fix the problem. The important thing is that by simply listening to someone we are doing something significant.

People will only talk when they want to and they will talk to the person they want to, in the same way that you identified earlier who you would talk to in a crisis. People do not always choose who they feel has the most knowledge or are the highest grade professionally; they more commonly choose the person that they feel most comfortable with, the person that they feel they connect with, and the person who is there at the right time. If you spend time just listening, having noticed and really seen that someone looks upset or worried, then you might say 'Would you like to tell me what's worrying you?' If they do not feel comfortable, they will not talk. When they do begin to talk, you cannot make the situation worse or make them more upset by just listening.

 ### Jenny's daughter Sarah

Erika was Jenny's regular carer and as Jenny became sicker, Erika's visits increased. Sarah, Jenny's daughter, was sometimes there but was still trying to keep on top of her job as a teacher while looking after her mum. One day Erika was leaving and saw Sarah sitting on the doorstep. She looked so sad. Erika knew she had to get to her next visit but chose to stop and sit next to Sarah. Erika said, 'You seem sad.' The two women sat for a moment and Sarah explained how tired she was and how hard it was to see her mum dying. Erika looked at Sarah and said, 'Do you need a hug?' – she said 'Yes.' That was what she most needed at that moment – nothing or no one could 'fix' the situation. Sarah felt a little better though; attention had been paid to her needs. Erika left and was still on time for her next visit.

Acknowledging

Sometimes you may notice that someone is looking upset, maybe tearful or looking sad. It is important that you acknowledge that you can see that the person is distressed. This can be just by sitting with them or saying, 'You seem upset, would you like to talk?' The person may not respond immediately. The temptation can be to leave but try not to rush away – just wait. If they can sense that you are there and that you want to help, then they are more likely to start to talk. It is important to acknowledge that the person has worries and seems anxious, frightened or scared. To be able to say 'I can see you look very worried today' or ' You seem very upset' is a powerful way of making a real connection with this person. They may well then share some feelings or concerns with you that will make a big difference to how they are going to cope with the time ahead. If you are still feeling worried about what to say, you could say, 'I can see that you have a lot on your mind today.'

These person-to-person interactions are very natural and often spontaneous and for some people just having this connection with another person is enough. Sometimes, though we have acknowledged the distress, it is evident that we are not the right person to take the conversation further. Sometimes it is appropriate to refer on to someone else. You could respond with a simple statement such as 'I am not sure I am the right person to talk to but I will find someone who is appropriate.' If, however, you are going to find someone else to talk to, it is important to make sure you go back and tell the person so that they are not left feeling even more alone and uncertain.

Being with someone

'Being with' someone can be immensely rewarding, offering the opportunity for them to share how they are feeling about dying with you. You may be surprised when you experience the difference that can be made by just listening to someone tell you how they are feeling. We are all responsible for supporting people we are looking after. Everyone is different but there are often shared concerns.

If you acknowledge what you see, that someone looks upset, worried or anxious, this will make a significant difference just by itself.

What concerns and worries may people approaching the end of life and their families have?

Think about what people approaching the end of their lives and those close to them may be concerned about. If it was someone close to you, what would your worries be?

It is normal to worry when we have to face difficult and challenging things in our lives. People worry about lots of different things but the primary, most significant concern can be different for different people. Take the examples of Maria and Jenny whose stories we are following through this book. Both say 'I am worried about dying.' We can assume the meaning of this question but unless we explore this with the person, we do not really know the true meaning behind the statement.

When Maria said she was worried about dying, it turns out that she was worried about becoming more breathless and that she would suffocate. But when Jenny said she was worried about dying, she was worried about how her family would manage without her. We have to remember we cannot assume what someone is worried about. We do not know what a person is worried about unless we ask. We have to listen to their concerns and explore them in order to find out. It takes 'detective work' – we need to follow all the clues and be prepared for things we might not expect.

When someone is dying, they may have concerns related to many aspects of their life, including their physical symptoms, emotions, family worries, financial or practical concerns or spiritual issues. As with Maria and Jenny, each person will have their particular unique worries.

Physical concerns

When someone is aware that they are going to die, an obvious question they may want to ask is 'What will it feel like to die?' This short question may be complicated with many different layers, so we should avoid making assumptions, presuming that we know what their main concern is. For some people it may be fear of choking to death, others may fear pain or breathlessness, some fear starving to death or being thirsty. If we are able to discover what their fear is, then there are often ways in which we can reassure them. For example, people rarely choke unless they have a specific underlying condition, so this may be something we can reassure them about.

Emotional concerns

People can say things like 'I feel very lost', 'I am not sure of anything', or 'Everything feels scary at the moment.' Feeling no longer in control of what is happening to you is one of the most difficult things to live with. Fear of the unknown makes people feel extremely anxious and can lead to feeling out of control. This lack of control can relate to what is happening to their bodies as well as their thoughts and feelings. When the person who is going to die slowly deteriorates, they may have to give up roles within the family and wider world such as employee, parent, child, partner. These things can wear down their sense of identity and cause emotional distress.

Spiritual concerns

When a person faces the end of their life, they can often reflect on their life and events within it. They may worry that they have done something wrong and in some way they deserve this diagnosis. They can believe that their lifestyle choices have led to a diagnosis of cancer or that their smoking is the primary cause of their stroke. This sense of guilt can also relate to other areas of the person's life. There may be unresolved issues with someone else and approaching death can bring these to the forefront of someone's mind. Equally, not everyone has regrets and some may feel they lived a good life and feel their life is complete.

A faith may also play a part in the dying person's spiritual concerns which may mean they want to speak to a faith leader. If religion is important to the person, you should have an understanding of what this means for them and how you can ensure they are able to practise the rituals of their faith. Some may question their faith, and its meaning for them at the end of their life.

Family concerns

What will happen to my family/children when I die? Can I talk with my family about what is happening and leave my thoughts and love in some way? This can lead to a feeling of real grief at the thought of leaving relatives and friends behind. They may experience a real sense of loss of role in society and in the family. For example, it can be hard to change from being the person who cared for everyone to becoming the one that is cared for. The relatives and carers will be having their own experience of this situation too. How will they cope without their loved one there for them? How can they best support them? Will they be strong enough to 'be there'?

Financial worries

Financial concerns can range from debt and inadequate income to needing to write a will. Housing issues that may be affected by the death can equally cause concern for both the person who is going to die and the family they leave behind.

Having listened to and explored their fears, we may be able to offer reassurance for some of them. It may be that we need to ask someone else to help us, for example, a social worker will be able to advise on housing problems.

When we consider all the different concerns and worries people may have, sometimes we can't reassure them. We don't have all the answers, but if we listen and explore their concerns it helps the person to feel that they have been heard. People we care for can feel very lonely and there is something very powerful about being truly heard.

Where should these conversations take place?

The conversations that we are discussing in this chapter are often difficult. We need to consider carefully the most appropriate place to have them. Would you feel comfortable talking about how you feel standing in a corridor or on a doorstep? Preparation is important – if the conversation is planned, then the most appropriate place should be found. It is important to establish where the person would feel most comfortable talking – would they prefer somewhere more private to share their thoughts or worries? Where will there be minimal interruptions? Practical issues such as the seating arrangements should also be considered. It is also important to establish who should be there.

Albert's bad news: when things don't go right

Albert was becoming increasingly unwell. He had a high temperature and a productive cough. The GP diagnosed a chest infection, the fourth one in as many months, and he was taken to hospital via an ambulance. Albert had dementia but moments of lucidity and was very scared. He pleaded with the ambulance crew to stay with him but they explained that they could not and he would be in 'good hands' with them. Jackie, his niece, arrived shortly afterwards. He was admitted to the medical assessment unit of the local hospital where a junior doctor explained that they could not keep treating these infections and advised that, in future, he should not be admitted and nature should take its course. Both Jackie and Albert were distressed by the news but more distressed by the way in which it was delivered. The doctor stood at the end of Albert's bed and their perception was that he shouted this significant news. They were given no privacy or time to absorb the information or any opportunity to ask questions. Bad news was bad enough but even more so when it was delivered in such a harsh way.

Conversations do not always go well but there are things that we can do to help them go as well as possible. This conversation could have easily been so different – the doctor could have drawn the curtains, gone to the bedside and allowed them more privacy.

> Think of where you work, where would be the most appropriate place for you to have a conversation with someone who is potentially distressed? Is there any way that you could improve this?

Confidentiality

If we are expecting people to tell us their concerns, we must respect their privacy and ensure that we maintain confidentiality. What they tell us is generally confidential and should not be shared with others without the person's consent. If we are told, for example, 'I really don't want to go back to hospital, I don't think there's any point', we should ask if we can share that information with our colleagues to try to ensure that their wishes are met. If, however, we feel that someone is at risk in some way, or will put others at risk, for example, if they say they are suicidal or want to harm someone else, then we have a duty to share the information with or without consent, and we should inform the person's GP and other professionals involved in providing their care. Often, however, the nature of these conversations is personal information about themselves or their families, about relationships. Rarely does this information need to be shared with others. If it is not relevant to their care, we should keep this sort of information private and confidential, no matter how interesting it is!

Positioning

If it is possible, sit down and have a similar chair to the person you are talking to so your heads are at the same level. This will really help for a couple of reasons. First, if you sit down, it gives the impression that you have time for that person. Second, it will help you and the other person to feel more comfortable in talking about difficult things. This will enhance what we call rapport.

The acronym *SURETY* (Stickley 2011) can be useful as a means of thinking how we can most effectively position ourselves and use our non-verbal as well as verbal skills:

>   *S* is for sitting at a comfortable angle.
>
>   *U* uncross legs and arms, have an open posture.
>
>   *R* is for remaining relatively relaxed.
>
>   *E* is for effective eye contact (not staring).
>
>   *T* is for touch.
>
>   *Y* use your intuition.

Time

Time is often used as an excuse as to why we don't start sensitive conversations – 'If I ask what the problem is, they may get upset' or 'I haven't got time to listen to everything that they have to say.' You may need to consider how you make the time. Some of these conversations will be incidental, they may happen when you least expect them – perhaps during personal care. This may be the first time that this person feels able to share their thoughts and worries with anyone, so it really is important that this moment is not missed. At times, we might feel pressured because of other work commitments or needing to be somewhere else but it can help both you and the person that you are talking to if you are clear about how much time you do have. It can be surprising how a really meaningful conversation can be very short.

What does good communication look like?

Good communication is made up of a number of skills. The use of the spoken word is just one of these.

Focused attention

This means giving all our concentration to the person who is speaking. This is not the same as staring at someone which might well make them feel very uncomfortable. It is more about being focused on what they are saying and how they are saying it. We communicate so much through our body and facial expressions, so we need to be aware of how someone is talking all the time. A deep sigh or someone looking down and looking particularity sad when they say something really needs to be noticed. All these ways that we communicate help to tell the story of how someone is feeling. We need to take in the whole picture.

If you were to watch a film with the sound turned off, you might well be able to make some of the story out but you might assume or make up bits too. So we need to hear and watch everything. If our attention were to drift away, this person might feel ignored or that their worries were not important or seemed silly. We need to really value their experience because it is theirs and this is how they feel. It does not matter if we think this does not make any sense or not, because this is their current experience.

Rapport

There are some people in your life to whom you will naturally feel more comfortable talking to than others, that you have a good rapport with. It may be that you have interests in common, you feel you can trust them, you have a shared past experiences or you simply know them really well. An important part of our communication can be the rapport that is built up.

Our first meeting can be very significant, as it will set the tone or mood for future contact. When we first meet someone, it will be important to get the introduction right, who you are and what your name is, alongside getting their name right. Creating an impression that you have time for that person can also help this experience of developing rapport. We have already talked about giving your focused attention to someone; add to this good eye contact and being aware of the other person's body language. A powerful tool can be to mirror the other person's body language, e.g. if they lean forward, then so do you. It really tells the person that you are present.

How we speak and our voice tone will also have a big impact on this feeling of being in unison. Imagine someone who is upset and feeling very sad. If you went to talk to them the way you might talk with friends if you were very excited about something, this would overwhelm this person and might make them move away from you. So begin talking quietly and sensitively, matching their mood and voice tone and this will enhance the feeling of being on the same wavelength. The people that we support can have this 'same wavelength' feeling about us, so may well choose you because you seem kind, approachable, and have time for them. If you match their mood and tone, the person you are talking to will be more comfortable with you, because you are listening and you have acknowledged that they look upset. Through your focused attention they will be more likely to share with you how they are feeling.

Think of a conversation that you have recently had with someone in your care. How do you think it went? Did you have rapport with the other person? How did they respond to you? List the skills that you used.

Active listening

There are many situations where we don't feel listened to. The other person may appear disinterested or just not taking in what we are trying to say. Listening is therefore a vital skill. Listening is different to questioning. Questioning will only give us answers to our questions, whereas listening will allow the person to tell us what is on their mind, or what their concerns are. But good listening is not just sitting there doing nothing; it is a highly skilled activity and is often referred to as 'active listening'.

Active listening is a skill that we can practise. It means listening in a way that encourages someone to continue telling us their story and then inviting them to say more. Some of the skills that we use for this are encouragement, silence, repetition and paraphrasing.

Encouragement

Encouragement can be shown through our facial expression, showing that we are listening and are interested in what the person is saying. We may nod our head, as if to say, 'Tell me more.' Sometimes we use short words to encourage them to continue, such as 'Uh-huh' or 'Mmm', and these short phrases show that you are listening and encourage the other person to continue.

Silence

Silence can be very powerful. If we are prepared to sit quietly with a person for a short while, it allows them to stay with the thoughts that are going around in their head. It gives them time to think and to formulate those thoughts before they choose to share them with us. A lot of people find silence uncomfortable, but it can be so important and is seldom uncomfortable for the person we are supporting. They are usually too busy thinking to even be aware of the silence.

If the silence does become uncomfortable, you may wish to try saying something like 'You seem to have a lot on your mind.'

Repetition or reflection

This is when we repeat the person's own words, like an echo. It encourages the person to continue telling us their story but without putting any pressure on them and allows them to follow the direction that they want to follow. For example, this is a conversation between Albert and his carer Bob when Albert was being helped to get ready for bed.

 ### Albert and his carer Bob

Bob: You're looking anxious, Albert.

Albert: Well, I'm just a bit worried.

Bob: Just a bit worried?

Albert: Well, yes, I'm just a bit worried about my niece, Jackie.

Bob: Just a bit worried?

Albert: You see, her husband's left her and she does not have a lot of money now, I think I need to look at my will again.

Bob: Would you like us to help you arrange to do that, Albert?

So by echoing what Albert said, Bob was able to find out what was on his mind and was then able to help him talk about it. Echoing encourages the person to continue telling us their story but without pressurising them.

Paraphrasing

Paraphrasing is the term used for summarising what we have heard by putting it into our own words. This lets the person know that we were listening and that we are acknowledging their concerns by using their own words to summarise what we have heard. This then gives the other person the opportunity to correct us or to expand on it further.

Equally, we can use the person's own words to summarise and to show that we have heard them. For example:

> **Albert:** *I am scared.*
>
> **Bob:** *You are scared.*

Picking up cues

When we begin to talk with people and want to hear their concerns, we will need to be attentive, listen and be a detective, all rolled into one. Sometimes people do not make what they are worried about very obvious. So we need to watch really carefully and look for clues and signs that would hint that there might be something else to talk about. Cues usually are a hint that there might be a larger worry hidden beneath what the person is talking about. Often people want to check us out to see if we are going to be a good person to have the conversation with. This may lead to them being able to talk about a deeper worry with you.

Cues can come in all sorts of ways. So we need to be very alert at all times during our conversation and watching for body language clues as well as really listening to what someone might be saying. The most obvious clue is when someone begins to cry, and we would be prepared to respond to this, as it is the most common sign that some-one is upset. There are other signs that might be more subtle like when someone sighs very heavily or looks down or goes quiet during a period of talking. Somebody may look more anxious by gripping their hands or hand wringing. It will take some practice to begin to notice these signs and for you to discover what is being expressed. This is when we need to explore a little deeper with the person about how they are feeling.

Let's consider some examples of what people might say where there might be a some deeper concerns.

Someone might say that they have been feeling very bothered by what's been happening. In this example, what do you think they might mean by the word 'bothered'? None of us are mind readers, so we need to ask. The easiest way to do this is to reflect back the word you want to know more about. By just saying the word 'bothered' and then leaving a pause, you will be surprised at how this will prompt them to say a bit more about what they could mean.

Another example might be 'I am not sure what to think about what is happening to me.' Again, this could have many hidden meanings so it is important to explore further or check out what it really means. So again we can repeat the words 'Not sure?' and then leave a pause. This then makes space for the person to begin to let you know what they are thinking. Once we can understand things from the other person's perspective or point of view we are in a much better position to be able to support the person.

Over the next few days, listen to conversations at home as well as at work and see how many cues you can notice, and think about what you could say that would encourage someone to tell you more.

Showing that we care

It is important that we not only care, but that we can show that we care, as then we are better able to support the person and those important to them. This may come more naturally to some people than others, but is an important skill that can be learnt. It is called empathy.

Empathy is more than sympathy. Sympathy is about expressing our sadness for another person's misfortune. Empathy is about communicating an understanding of the other person's feelings and the situation that they are in and communicating this understanding back to them in a sensitive and helpful way. To understand another person's predicament, we have to use all the skills that we have talked about. We will use our active listening; we will explore the cues that we are given, and we will paraphrase and summarise to show that we have heard and to check that our understanding is correct. It is also important to note that we can demonstrate empathy in the words that we use such as: 'You are going through a lot at the moment' or 'This is really hard.' We should use the words carefully and feel comfortable saying them. Very rarely do the words said empathetically and with sensitivity come across as trite.

Jenny's good days and bad days

Jenny is visited weekly by her district nurse Beth, and Beth is always impressed at how upbeat Jenny is. Despite becoming increasingly weak, she always has a project on the go. She has decided that she wants to make memory boxes for her three grandchildren.

Beth arrives to find Jenny clutching a photo of her granddaughter and crying quietly. Beth does not know what to do. She puts her hand on Jenny's shoulder and says: 'This must be really hard for you.' The short silence is broken by Jenny agreeing that it is but it is something she wants and needs to do. She talks about how special her grandchildren are. Beth listens and then Jenny wipes away her tears and they get on with the matter in hand.

Beth did not know what to say but that one simple statement gave Jenny permission to say more. Jenny and Beth were 'connected'. Beth also put her hand on Jenny's shoulder, showing empathy through touch. It is not always appropriate to touch someone in this way but we can still show empathy though our body language, by moving closer to someone or leaning forward perhaps.

Non-verbal communication

To express our understanding back shows the person who is dying that we understand and that we care about what they are going through. To do this, we use not only the spoken language but the non-spoken language as well. This is called non-verbal communication, or body language.

Good non-verbal communication can sometimes say things that a thousand words would never be able to say. Sometimes there are no words to say, but being able to sit quietly with someone and to hold their hand can mean so much.

Touch can be a sensitive issue, and is affected by culture, experience and preference. In general, it should feel natural, and if it feels forced it probably isn't right. We touch people when we wash them, when we help them get dressed, and when we are helping them up from a chair. We also use touch when we are comforting them when they are upset or when we are giving them a hug to share their happiness. It can express an acceptance, closeness and an understanding; but we need to really watch and notice any sort of response and if we sense that they are feeling awkward or may have been offended, we must stand back and perhaps even apologise. Facial expression can show that we care and that we are sensitive to the person's predicament. We don't have to have been through the same thing as someone in order to be empathic, but it is necessary to be able to see things from their point of view. By using some of these skills, we will be able to do that and be able to show them that we care.

What happens if we do not listen to someone's worries of concerns?

When we are supporting or looking after someone, it is very tempting to only talk about what we feel comfortable talking about. It can feel easier to focus on practical issues or stay on lighter topics or chit chat. These conversations are also important and have their place. However, it is important not to avoid conversation that makes us feel less comfortable. If we do not talk about how people are feeling or follow up on the cues about some stronger emotional concerns, this will lead to someone feeling more distressed and isolated. This could lead to people becoming anxious or depressed. It is important that we spend time with someone so we can encourage them to talk through their worries rather than letting it all fester and brew up into something much deeper and darker. When you encourage someone to open up to you about their feelings, then confirming that you have heard what they have said and its significance, is really important for them. Sharing how they feel can let someone feel better and less anxious.

How to respond to 'difficult' questions?

Sometimes we can be asked a very difficult question, out of the blue, and it can feel like a real challenge to know how to respond. It will be important to think about why someone is asking this question right now. We must respond with honesty and we must not pretend we know something when we don't. We must also be careful that we don't harm someone by giving them answers that they are not ready to hear and would cause distress. It is important to think things through before answering immediately, so having a structure might help. The worst thing that we can do is ignore the question.

The sort of questions that people may ask could include:

- How am I going to die?
- Will I be able to walk again?
- Will I have pain?

Before answering any of these, we first need to find out what the person already knows, whether they really want to know the answer, and why are they asking the question. For example, in answer to the question: 'How long have I got?' First, it is important to establish why they are asking the question – have they overheard a conversation or misinterpreted something? A simple response could be 'Why do you ask that?' which will clarify but also help us detect how much the person wants to know. Their response could be that they thought that they had only had a few days left to live. If they say this, we may then be able to tell them that we think they could be right or wrong. In this way we avoid giving them unexpected or unwanted news, as they have been leading the conversation.

Some of these conversations can be hard. We may not always feel qualified to continue, but by asking whether they want to know or not, we avoid doing harm by telling those things they did not want to know. Figure 4.1 is a flow chart for answering difficult questions.

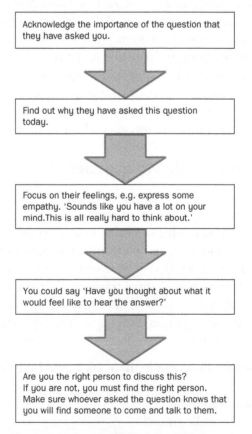

Figure 4.1 Flow chart of answering difficult questions

Maria and her carer Shazia

A conversation between Maria and her carer Shazia went like this:

Maria: *How am I going to die?*

Shazia: *What makes you ask that, Maria?*

Maria: *Well, I don't want to choke to death.*

Shazia: *That's not what happens, Maria, it is usually very peaceful.*

Maria: *Will I go to hospital if I get another chest infection?*

Shazia: *What do you want to happen?*

Maria: *Well, I don't think there is much point really, I'm not going to get better, I'd rather stay at home.*

Shazia: *Is that something that you would like me to tell the doctor? They could come and talk about it with you some more.*

In this way the conversation has been led by Maria and has been taken at a pace that she is comfortable with. No distress has been caused and she is feeling reassured and supported.

Be aware, there are some common pitfalls to avoid:

- *Assumptions*: Sometimes we assume that we know what people are thinking. Isn't it obvious? We think she must be worried about pain. Well, it is not always obvious. She may be worried about her children and not about pain. If we check things out with the person, we can understand things from their perspective. We have to sensitively explore what their worries and concerns really are so that we can understand them better and no distress is caused.
- *Not ignoring*: When caring for people's physical support needs, washing and feeding for example, we are in an ideal position to listen to the person's worries and in so doing, be able to support them through difficult times. The physical closeness that we have while caring for them often makes people felt safe and secure and so able to share their concerns. They often give us cues that show they want to talk to us, for example fidgeting, sighing or crying. If we ignore this, they will think we don't want to listen. If we comment on these signals and explore them further, they see that we are interested and are more likely to share

further worries with us. So no matter how busy we are, we should remain alert for these signals. If we really are unable to make time now, acknowledge that you see this person is upset, say you will return and when, and, most importantly, come back when you say you will. Sometimes circumstances and time commitments mean that we have to leave someone distressed. If this does happen, it is vital that the distress of the person is acknowledged and that the person knows when you or someone else will return. The following statements may help: 'This is really upsetting for you', 'I have to go now but will be back in two hours' or 'I am sorry to see you so upset. I need to go now but will be back in half an hour so we can talk then.'

- *Boundaries*: It is important that we think about the relationship that we have with the person that we are caring for. If we are employed to look after this person, then this is a professional relationship and we need to behave in an appropriate way, within boundaries. This is so to protect both ourselves and the people that we are supporting. Some of the relationships that we have with the people can be over months or even years; this though does not make them our friend. We are very friendly, kind and supportive but this person is not part of our private life. This means that we need to be clear about how much we share of ourselves, our family and our worries at work. We have talked about building a rapport with the person we are supporting but this does not mean bringing our home life into work. We need to look after ourselves and make sure that we do not get over-involved as this would impact on the way we are able to look after someone. Looking after people can be stressful so it is important we leave work at work. **Chapter 11** discusses why this is important and includes suggestions on what may help you do this.

Sometimes it's hard to get the balance right for the people we are supporting. Some people can feel lonely and want to know a lot about the people caring for them – what their families are doing, holiday plans, and so on. We must decide how much we want to share and draw our own boundaries. If we are being employed to support someone, the balance of conversations should be about the person not us.

When we care, we sometimes feel sad – and that's OK. Sometimes it's OK to shed tears with the person we are looking after, but we have to remember that it is our job to look after them and we shouldn't be so upset that they feel they have to look after us.

Multicultural awareness and sensitivities

We live in a multicultural society and need to be aware that people live and act in different ways. When we first meet with people from different ethnic backgrounds we need to think about their language skills, whether shaking hands is acceptable and normal for them, whether they are comfortable to see male or female professionals, how their name is pronounced and how they wish to be addressed, and what rituals and traditions need to be observed at the end of life. The answers to these questions can be explored though gentle conversation with the person being cared for and those close to them. If there is a language barrier, we may need to adapt how we communicate, using short and clear sentences. We should only ask one question at a time and aim to give information in small chunks, checking that the person has understood frequently. This principle of chunking and checking is useful in all our communications but can be particularly helpful when we are speaking to someone who has a different language. We also need to show respect for all individuals, no matter what their background, and to be aware of our own shortcomings, for example, not being able to speak their language.

Communicating when language is a barrier can be a demanding situation and we need patience and compassion to do this well. We need to think carefully about the language we are using and the way in which we are speaking.

Physical barriers to communication

The same principles can be applied to those whose language skills are affected by strokes, learning disability or physical ailments such as breathlessness, for example. We need to take time and be patient and, if necessary, ask for help. We may need to ask for an interpreter or for someone who can use sign language. Some people who find it difficult to speak, for example, after a stroke, may find it easier to write things down on a pad. Others may prefer to use electronic devices and the speech and language therapist can advise on this.

Empowerment

When people come and live in a group of any sort, we tend to give them a name as well as their own, e.g. patient, resident, client. This means that they lose some of their sense of self-determination and may feel disempowered. They will begin to feel a loss of control of their daily life. Imagine your own life for a moment and think about how many decisions and choices that you make every day. From big things about relationships and what job you might like to do, to the very small things like what time you get out of bed and what you choose to wear. You are in a position to take charge of many of your daily activities.

Think about the people that you are supporting compared to yourself. How many active choices or decisions are they able to make? If we were to lose our own self-determination, we would soon become extremely fed up, frustrated and depressed.

Add into this mix how you are feeling about where you are, who comes to see you, or not, and if you do not fully understand what your immediate future might be like, because you are slowly dying.

Throughout this chapter we have looked at a number of skills that we can use and approaches we can take when talking to someone. All of these will, we hope, help the person we are caring for feel more empowered – help them to feel a bit more in charge of their lives. To make people feel like the person they have always been. If they feel powerless and are worried or distressed about something for a lot of the time, this will really have an impact on their mood.

If we want each person to be in charge of as much of their life as they are able to, we need to talk with them and discover what this sounds and feels like. Feeling out of control of your life is a really horrible place to be. We need to advocate for people or support any changes so that they can feel more in charge. If someone is really worried, fretting and anxious about their immediate future, this will take away from any feeling of being in control.

Talking to people about dying: things to remember

- People choose who they talk to, who they share concerns with.
- Say what you see – if someone looks upset, worried, annoyed, they probably are, so acknowledge it.
- Acknowledging the feeling is not the same as resolving the problem.
- Lack of time can be an excuse not to listen, but listening and giving someone your time is important.
- If you don't know what to say, listen, explore and listen again.

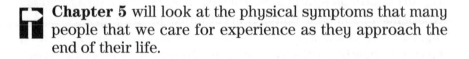 **Chapter 5** will look at the physical symptoms that many people that we care for experience as they approach the end of their life.

What are the common physical symptoms at the end of life and how can we help?

Christine Linley, Belinda Hitchens and Karen Cook

When many people think about dying, they are frightened that they will suffer difficult **symptoms.** This fear may be based on a previous experience of someone dying, films or books portraying slow lingering deaths or simply a lack of knowledge. Some people approaching the end of their life will suffer multiple symptoms, others will experience none. This chapter will:

- identify the common physical symptoms experienced as the end of life approaches;
- focus on how you assess the person and recognise if they are experiencing physical symptoms;
- offer suggestions to help you support the person experiencing symptoms and how you can help manage these.

The focus of this chapter is an explanation of each of the symptoms with the emphasis being on what *you* can do to help. Some symptoms may require the use of medications and some of the key drugs and how they are administered will be discussed at the end of the chapter. Other non-physical symptoms will be discussed in **Chapter 6.**

The symptoms considered in this chapter are:

- pain and discomfort;
- shortness of breath or breathlessness;
- feeling sick and being sick;
- dry or sore mouth;
- changes to bowel habits;

- appetite changes and problems with eating;
- poor mobility and loss of independence.

How do we know if a person is experiencing a symptom?

Some symptoms will cause more anxiety to some people than others. The way in which the symptom is experienced can also vary – agony for one person could be moderate discomfort for another. We can never fully know what the person is experiencing until we assess them. This may be by what we see or what they tell us, but most probably by a combination of both. Until we find out from the person how they are affected we are really only guessing. Some people may feel they can manage a certain symptom at a certain level while another symptom, which may appear to be minor to us, may have a huge impact on someone and their quality of life.

Assessing symptoms

Assessment is a vital part of helping to manage a person's symptoms and it is important to find out what the symptom feels like to that person and how it is affecting their life. For some symptoms this may seem obvious. The person may be grimacing, crying out, rubbing a part of their body, they may be unable to stand without help, may experience difficulty catching their breath after minor activity or generally look uncomfortable and restless. Other symptoms may be more difficult to recognise or observe. For example, how would you know if someone was feeling nauseated or low in mood? Symptom assessment tools are available to assess and record the degree of the symptom that someone may experience. A tool may be a series of questions, it may be more visual asking the individual or the person caring for them to plot the degree of the symptom on a line from 'not present' to 'worst ever'. When recording a symptom it is vital that we all use the same measures. Visual assessment tools include stools charts that have pictures of various types of faeces – soft, constipated, etc. so that everyone knows that what they are recording is consistent. Assessment tools can be used to record severity but also risk. The Waterlow score, for example, is a widely acknowledged assessment tool looking at the risk of someone developing a **pressure sore**. Questions asked include ones related to the person's size, mobility, nutritional status, how likely they are to develop a pressure sore and any changes that should be made to their care as a result of the assessment of their risk.

Many symptoms, however, we assess best by knowing the person that we are looking after – the person may seem 'different', not their usual self. In this way everyone should be involved in assessing symptoms, it is not only senior or specific health professionals. A large part of assessment is being aware of any differences or changes to a person – this can be done by anyone.

Jenny's pain

Jenny is experiencing some pain related to her cancer. When she first experienced this, the pain was intermittent, happening every now and again. Everyone she came into contact with asked her whether she had any pain – her family, her GP, even the hospital consultant. She explained that, yes, she did, but that it was OK – she could manage it. Jenny began to wonder why this was such an issue for everyone when she didn't feel it was a problem. Jenny was more concerned about the fact that she was feeling nauseated – not all the time but definitely when she travelled to the many different hospital appointments. No one asked if she had any other concerns, they were so focused on pain that she didn't raise it.

As you read through this chapter, think about how you might check whether the person is experiencing any symptoms. How would they look?, what might they say?, what might you observe?, what questions would you ask?, how would you know what was important to that person?

Pain and discomfort

Pain should always be viewed from the perspective of the person experiencing it. In short, pain is what the person says it is. Each of us will experience pain in our own unique way. This is coloured by our own past knowledge and experiences, that pain we have experienced before in our lives, whether we have cared for a loved one who has experienced pain, how effective pain medication has been in the past, and what we associate pain with. This is the same for the people we are caring for. Some people may experience 'total pain' – this is suffering that affects all of a person's physical, psychological, social, spiritual and practical struggles. Total pain is the idea that people don't just experience pain because of a physical problem, but that it is also related to other issues in their life.

Think about a time when you have had a physical pain that you have experienced more than once, for example, a headache. What other things may affect your headache? Would you feel differently if you were in a positive or a low mood? Would you feel differently if you were anxious or bored?

Some of the people that we look after will describe discomfort rather than pain, and they may feel they can cope with a certain level of discomfort, for example, Jenny. This is why person-centred assessment and management of pain are important. Assessing pain and other symptoms should be done regularly, not just when the person mentions their symptom; and it should be documented so that there is a record of the assessment, what action was taken and the impact of this action, that is, did it help?

Some of the questions that should be asked include:

- Does the person look comfortable? Is the person telling you that they feel uncomfortable?
- Do we know what is causing the pain? Is the pain related to another problem, for example, constipation, indigestion, immobility, etc.?
- How does the individual describe their pain? Is it a constant ache, intermittent, a dull sensation, hot/burning? If the pain is a hot, burning pain, would a cold pack help?
- Is there anything that eases their pain/discomfort or that makes it worse? Is one position more comfortable than another? Does movement worsen the pain? What about coughing, laughing, having a bowel motion, eating or feeling worried?
- What helps the person deal with their pain and discomfort? What has worked for them before? For example, does heat or cold help? Does gentle massage help?

These are simple questions that can help provide a picture of the individual's pain. Once we understand the individual's experience of pain and discomfort, we can work with them to try to lessen this. Pain assessment tools are useful documents which can help us to assess and record the details of someone's pain. If they are used regularly, they can indicate if the treatment we are giving is helping, or if we need to consider something different. Most people that we care for have a team of people looking at them, so the use of such tools can help us ensure that the person gets continuity of care.

Some tools ask the person to plot the degree of their pain on a scale of 1 to 10, with 1 being no pain and 10 being the worst pain ever. Others are based on a drawing of the human body, back and front, and the person is asked to mark or point on the diagram where the pain is, whether it moves anywhere and, if so, where and how would they describe the type of pain? A list of descriptive words can also help the person explain what the pain is like – burning, stabbing, throbbing, shooting, for example.

These symptom assessment tools can be useful, but rely on the person telling us what they are feeling. Sometimes the person who is dying will be unable to communicate by speaking, or have limited ability to understand, comprehend or remember what they have experienced. This may be relevant to those with communication difficulties, for example, someone who has suffered a stroke and has difficulty with speech (dysphasia); someone who has dementia, short-term memory problems or learning difficulties. There are pain assessment scores that can be used for these different groups. One example is the **Abbey Pain Scale**. The scale is completed by a healthcare professional or carer who is familiar with the individual and can rate changes in their behaviour which may indicate that they are experiencing pain or discomfort. This is used when the individual being assessed is unable to think through or verbally communicate their experience of pain.

Find out about different pain assessment tools that may be available to use where you work and relevant to the people you care for. Why not try going online and searching for pain assessment tools or familiarise yourself with the ones your organisation uses? Have a go at using them. Are they helpful?

Albert's experience of pain

Albert has had a stroke and that, together with his advancing dementia, makes communication difficult.

The care home staff have noticed that he is 'not himself'. He seems more distracted than usual, frowning and rubbing his tummy. His appetite has never been good, but he is now refusing all food. On closer inspection his abdomen appears distended or swollen. He ignores the question 'Are you in pain?' but when the word ache is used, he nods. Those caring for Albert recall that this has happened before. It is discovered that he is constipated – this is easily resolved with laxatives and Albert returns to his normal self.

Those caring for Albert knew him well enough to know that something was not right. He could not say that he was in pain, but there was something causing him distress.

Breakthrough pain

Despite being given regular medication to control their pain some people may experience **breakthrough pain.** This kind of pain can spontaneously occur or can be incident-related, for example, it happens when the client moves, coughs, or has a dressing changed. Avoidance of the activity can be a means of resolving the pain, but it is not always possible if they get pain when standing or using the commode, etc. For these types of pain, it is invaluable for the client to have an immediate-release painkiller available, which they can safely take with their regular medications. In the example, Albert's pain was assessed, the cause treated (and resolved) and recorded. In different circumstances, when the cause is not so easily resolved, it is more difficult.

Cast your mind back to your headache that we considered earlier. It may be that painkillers would help you, but we often think of doing something else first – fresh air perhaps or maybe you need to drink more water. This is equally true of the people whom we are looking after.

Avoiding a particular painful position may help reduce the pain. If the pain is intermittent and related to a particular movement or activity, reducing the number of times that particular movement or activity is carried out in one day may help. A physiotherapist or **occupational therapist** may help to discover different techniques or equipment that may be helpful. **Chapter 3** gives details of the different people involved in care who could help with this. Techniques could include re-positioning for comfort, planning an activity with the person, helping them to pace any painful activity and to prioritise those activities which are most important over those that could be minimised. A hospital or community-based physiotherapist or occupational therapist service should be available in your local area.

Managing pain without the use of medication

Knowing the person will help you to think about things that have helped in the past. You may, for example, know ways that help them relax. If you don't know them well, asking them may help gather the same information. Some people may benefit from complementary therapies. Aromatherapy massage, reflexology, acupuncture, hypnotherapy can all be useful in the management of pain. While most of these require a specialist to deliver the therapy, there are some simple things that any of us can do. You may like to suggest a simple relaxation technique.

Relaxation

Here are two simple relaxation sessions that can be read aloud to help someone to relax. It may help to record them so that the person can listen to them whenever they wish.

Muscle relaxing and breathing

1.   *Sit in a comfortable chair.*
2.   *Begin by squeezing your toes up or crunch them up really tightly, as much as you can.*
3.   *Take a deep breath and release the tension from your toes. You are now going to imagine tensing and then releasing muscles in your body moving upwards throughout your body.*

4.   So start with your toes, tense them, release them.
5.   So now tense your calves, release, and breathe out.
6.   Tense your thighs, release, and breathe out.
7.   Hold in your tummy and then release and breathe out.
8.   Pull your shoulders up to reach your ears and hold the tension and then release and breathe out.
9.   Scrunch up all your facial muscles with your eyes closed and then release the tension and breathe out.
10. Make a tight fist of your hands and tense your arms and then release and breathe out.
11. Now, focusing on a soft feeling throughout your body and breathing calmly and rhythmically, stay in this relaxed place for as long you are able.

Visualising a positive experience

1.   Sit in a comfortable chair or lie down. Close your eyes and focus on your breathing.
2.   Be aware of your breath slowly moving in and out of your body, and, as you breathe out, imagine that all your unwanted tension is leaving your body.
3.   Think of a place, it might be real or it might be imagined.
4.   Imagine yourself there – it could be by the sea or in a lovely garden somewhere. It might be the perfect holiday destination.
5.   Concentrate on being at that place – where are you sitting or lying?, what you are wearing?, what is the weather like?, can you feel the sun or the wind on your face?
6.   Focus your breathing and be aware of yourself beginning to feel really, really relaxed. Stay in this place in your imagination for as long as you would like.
7.   Then slowly return to where you are, feeling refreshed and relaxed.

Another helpful activity to help someone to relax is hand massage. This can be as simple as gently stroking their hand using lotions or oils. This can be soothing and can help refocus the person's mind on something other than their discomfort. It can also be taught to family members, who can sit with their relative with purpose, and can give both parties great comfort.

For some people, the one thing that can help the most may be as simple as distraction. Try to think of activities available that may help refocus the person's attention on something other than the pain, for example, television, music, conversation or a change of scenery.

Find out how people in your care can get access to advice, equipment (if needed) and therapy. Do they have to pay for it? Do they have to be referred via their GP? What other services are available in your area, for example, physiotherapy, aromatherapy?

Shortness of breath or breathlessness

Shortness of breath or breathlessness is the unpleasant and often frightening experience of being aware of difficulty breathing. The sensation of breathlessness can be common in people entering the last part of their lives. Breathlessness can occur for lots of different reasons, though it may not always be related to a particular problem with their lungs or airway. Shortness of breath in the last weeks and months of someone's life may be as result of a number of things including:

● lung conditions/disease
● build-up of fluid (oedema)
● secretions in the lungs
● build-up of fluid in the chest cavity (pleural effusion)
● weakened muscles
● low levels of red blood cells (anaemia)
● pain
● clots in the lungs (pulmonary emboli)
● anxiety or panic
● a general deterioration in a person's condition.

Just as with pain, the sensation of breathlessness is individual; a person may not look overtly short of breath but for them their experience is one of difficulty breathing. As listed above, shortness of breath has a physical element, however there is often a strong psychological element, particularly for people approaching the end of life, as they can associate worsening breathlessness with their illness getting worse. The more frightened the person becomes about their breathing, often the more breathless they will become.

Think about a person you have cared for who complains of difficulty catching their breath. How did they look? What helped them?

Once again knowledge of the person is helpful. Some people we look after will have experienced shortness of breath before. It may be helpful to find out and record what has helped them in the past. This should be before or after the person is experiencing breathlessness and not when their shortness of breath is most acute. Here are some ways to support those who are experiencing feelings of breathlessness. These are things that will help the person to maintain as much control, and we hope independence, as possible. In **Chapter 9** we will think about the changes in a person's breathing that may occur as they approach death.

Breathing techniques

Encouraging a person to focus more on the 'out breaths' can be helpful. People who are breathless tend to focus on the 'in breaths' feeling desperate to get air in while neglecting the 'out breath', and hyperventilation can occur. Hyperventilation is the experience of an excessive increase in quantity of breaths, often shallow. Being encouraged to extend the out breath or sigh as they breathe out can be helpful.

Position

It may be that the person finds a sitting position more comfortable. If sitting in a chair, it can be helpful to lean forward onto a table with a pillow on top. This will allow the person to lean forwards and rest their forearms on the pillow, effectively fixing their ribcage in position so assisting with breathing. This can also be achieved for people in bed with an over-bed table.

It can be helpful to have a hospital bed to allow the person to be positioned more easily in bed. A hospital bed can be profiled to enable the bed to support the person in their most comfortable position, which could be with their head elevated in an armchair position or enabling their legs to bend with the bed at the person's knees. In a standard bed, propping a person up with pillows or using a back rest (which can be provided by an occupational therapist or district nurse) can help. Having a small pillow in the small of the back can help open up the ribcage. Arms should be supported on pillows.

Air movement

Using a hand-held fan, an electric fan or open window to help circulate the air can be helpful. The fan should be held 6 inches away from the middle of the face, allowing the air to blow towards the top lip and around the sides of the nose. Alternatively, being positioned by an open window or electric fan where there is a breeze can also help to relieve the experience of breathlessness. Moving the chair or bed nearer to an open window or an electric fan may also help.

Taking your time (pacing)

The essential activities that we all do every day (or activities of daily living) may be more difficult if a person is experiencing breathlessness. There are many practical things a person can do to reduce the effort involved in everyday tasks. They may need your support and encouragement to help achieve these; advise them not to do all the tasks at once but to rest in between. Some practical suggestions are:

- to sit rather than stand whenever possible;
- to breathe in when reaching up and breathe out when bending down;
- to think about clothing, for example, having slip-on shoes and clothes which fasten at the front;
- to use an electric toothbrush and an electric shaver;
- to consider a walking aid, for example, a stick or frame;
- to limit time spent talking – concentrate on talking about what is important to the person;
- to ensure the room is well ventilated;
- to limit the use of the stairs – maybe only down in the morning and up at bedtime – a commode, if no downstairs toilet, may help or a chair positioned halfway on the landing.

Reassurance and talking

The person may benefit from talking about their fears about breathlessness. They may also benefit from understanding a little more about the mechanism of breathing and identifying the things that worsen their sensation of breathlessness. A greater understanding of what is happening, and is likely to happen, can help the person identify what will help them; for example, the involvement of a physiotherapist may help.

Relaxation

The use of relaxation techniques can help with managing breathlessness. The experience of breathlessness can be frightening and anxiety may make the breathlessness worse. Helping the person to remain as calm as possible may also help. Earlier on in the chapter we gave an example of relaxation techniques. The person can use the exercise on their own or work though it with someone else.

An occupational therapist can give advice on daily living activities and any equipment or alternative ways of doing things to avoid breathless episodes.

Maria is short of breath

Maria has had heart failure for three years and her condition is getting worse. It used to be that she was just short of breath when she exerted herself. She can no longer lie flat so sits propped up with pillows in the new bed that the district nurse ordered. She says that the worst thing is that it stops her talking – her favourite pastime! The district nurse visited her and her family bought her a fan that she could hold by her face– she likes this because it is something that she can control, she feels like she is losing control of so much at the moment.

Feeling sick and being sick

Nausea and vomiting can be common symptoms at the end of life and can reduce the quality of life. For some, the feeling of nausea can be worse as it can lead to feeling constantly unwell. The occasional vomit can help some people to feel relief and so they can tolerate this. This will be an individual experience and so would need to be discussed and assessed with the individual. Although the experience of nausea and/or vomiting is unpleasant, there is much you can do to help alleviate it.

Talking through the problem with the person may help establish why they are feeling or being sick, help discover what is making the situation worse, recognise what to avoid and identify what has helped in the past. Helping people understand what is happening and why can help alleviate anxiety which can help with feelings of nausea.

> Think about a time when you have been with someone who was either nauseated or vomiting. What helped them? What made their symptoms worse? And was there anything they did to help themselves?

Nausea and vomiting are controlled in the brain by an area known as the Vomiting Centre. The Vomiting Centre receives signals from triggers located in several different areas within the body, including the stomach and ear. Senses such as smell, taste and pain can also trigger the signals, as can emotions such as anxiety. **Chapter 6** will look in more detail about anxiety. For this reason, assessment is essential as effective treatment depends on the underlying causes being identified.

What can cause nausea and vomiting?

Nausea and vomiting can be caused by many different reasons, and often a combination of triggers is involved. Whatever the cause, it can be a distressing and debilitating experience.

Possible causes of nausea and vomiting at the end of life may be:

- chemical imbalances such as high levels of blood calcium or potassium;
- the consequences of liver or renal failure;
- treatment-related, for example, chemotherapy or radiotherapy for cancer;
- the drugs we offer people for other symptoms can often themselves lead to nausea, for example, pain-relieving medication, such as morphine-based drugs, commonly cause nausea, however, other medication such as anti-inflammatories, antibiotics and iron can also be a cause;

- nausea and/or vomiting can be a sign of another condition such as urine infection or constipation;
- it may also be a sign that the person has developed a more serious condition such as bowel obstruction or a blockage in the bowel, which prevents the movement of material along the length of the gut.

As we have seen in this chapter, many physical symptoms also have a psychological element. Some people will feel sick when they are anxious, others may experience anticipatory nausea or vomiting – when the person expects to feel sick or vomit in particular circumstances, for example, when they eat certain foods, or take certain medicines, such as chemotherapy treatments.

Although medications may be helpful and will be discussed later in this chapter, often there may be some simple things which you can do to help a person to manage the sensation of nausea and possibly reduce episodes of vomiting. Reducing the vomiting will in turn increase dietary intake which can be an issue for many at the end of life.

Odour

Food can be a trigger for nausea and vomiting, and you can probably remember when this was true for you. It may be the sight and/or the smell of food that can be a trigger. Strong food smells which may make a person feel sick should be avoided. It is also worth noting that chilled foods tend to smell less than hot foods.

Some people feel bloated in conjunction with feeling sick and peppermints or peppermint water can help certain individuals.

It is worth considering where the person is eating. It may help if you create a calm environment where someone can eat the amount they want, at a pace that suits them.

Many of the people that we are caring for benefit from small frequent meals or snacks. Presentation is important, make the food look as attractive as possible and avoid large plates of food which can be off-putting. Consider foods containing ginger, for example, biscuits, tea or non-alcoholic ginger beer as some report that taking food and drink containing ginger helps reduce the experience of nausea. Be aware that not everyone likes the taste of these strong flavours. Encourage the person to sip drinks slowly. Think also of practical issues, such as their positioning in the chair or bed, sitting as upright as possible for meals and drinks. Also make sure water, bowls and tissues are close at hand in case the person has to vomit.

Unpleasant smells from, for example, colostomy bags, bowel motions or wounds should be masked if possible. Simple solutions may be ventilating the room or using an **aroma stone** which can add a scent to the room. Scents that can help include peppermint, lavender, lemon grass and citrus-based smells.

Complementary therapies

The use of 'sea-bands', bands worn on the wrists that apply pressure to acupressure points in the wrist may be helpful for the sensation of motion sickness. Acupuncture may also help, but would require a trained acupuncturist. As previously discussed, essential oils on an aroma stone or electric vaporiser can be used to disguise the smell but can also help the person to relax and reduce the anxiety, particularly if nausea happens when the person anticipates the sensation of sickness. Some people may benefit from listening to relaxation recordings or taking part in activities that they find relaxing, such as yoga.

Dry or sore mouth

Many people approaching the end of their life experience a dry or painful mouth. Although this may seem a minor problem to those giving the care, it can have a major impact on those suffering from these symptoms. It can affect how much they are able to eat and drink and even how well they can communicate.

Why mouth problems are common

Healthy people produce around 1.5 litres of saliva a day. This keeps the mouth moist and healthy. Saliva also has antibacterial properties which helps to prevent infection in the mouth. When people are unwell they often produce less saliva and this is made worse by several other possible factors, that may include:

● finding it hard to eat and drink, perhaps due to other symptoms, such as feeling sick or weak;

- medications may make their mouth drier, for example, it is a common side-effect of painkillers;
- certain treatments, such as chemotherapy or radiotherapy (to head and neck area), can make the mouth sore and dry;
- people who are unwell may find it difficult to care for their own mouth.

Ways to help improve a dry/sore mouth

Good basic mouth care is very important and the first thing to try. This may mean encouraging the person to help themselves by brushing their teeth. If the person is unable to care for their own mouth, it is essential that you help with this. Teeth should be brushed twice a day. This should include gently brushing of the tongue particularly if the tongue is coated. Using a soft toothbrush is often helpful, for example, a toothbrush designed for a baby or young child may be more comfortable for the person involved.

Dry mouth

Here are some other things you could offer to help someone suffering with a dry mouth:

- taking frequent sips of water, or any drink that they enjoy;
- sucking ice chips, ice lollies or frozen fruit juice may help;
- sipping fruit juices such as pineapple may help;
- ginger or lemon-flavoured drinks and foods can help boost saliva production in some people;
- using a lip balm or petroleum jelly to keep their lips supple;
- replacement saliva sprays and gels can be helpful and would need to be prescribed.

Sore mouth

A sore mouth can be very uncomfortable and stop someone eating, drinking, talking and taking medication. There are, however, some simple things that you can do to help. Keeping the mouth moist and clean is essential. Try to ensure that food is soft and bland, such as mashed potato or scrambled eggs. You could also try softening other foods with gravy or another sauce. If hot food hurts, let it cool down or offer cool or cold alternatives such as ice cream, jelly or yogurt. Try to avoid things that can make their mouth hurt – common triggers include citrus drinks and foods (e.g. orange, lemon), alcohol and tobacco, crunchy or spicy foods.

Underlying problems should always be treated where possible and you may need to seek medical advice if the person you are caring for has:

- difficulty in eating or swallowing;
- infection in the mouth and throat – a common fungal infection is thrush (or oral candida) and will require treatment with antibiotics;
- painful sores in their mouth or on the lips, for example, ulcers, can be made less painful with local anaesthetic agents which can be bought from a chemist. Cold sores may need specific cream application.

Regular mouthwashes can also be useful; some alcohol-based mouthwashes, however, can dry the mouth out more. Mouthwashes may also feel very strong and astringent if someone has a sore mouth, so some care needs to be taken to check that this is not the case. For some people, a mouthwash with a local anaesthetic may help soothe the soreness – this may need a prescription.

Difficulties cleaning Albert's mouth

Albert now needs help with all aspects of his personal care. He used to clean his own teeth but that has now stopped. One carer suggests that if 'he puts up a fight, it is not worth bothering.' Her colleagues quickly challenge her and explain why she is so wrong. Albert should be treated with dignity and respect, they tell her and that means attending to all his care needs, however difficult. He is drinking less and less and it is therefore even more important that his mouth is kept clean for his comfort and to avoid fungal infection or decay. Cleaning his teeth also means that his mouth can be assessed on a regular basis and any deterioration managed. The dementia nurse specialist visited some time ago and suggested standing behind Albert as he sits on a dining room chair, supporting his head on your body and cleaning his teeth from behind him. He seems to accept this and now the carer will not forget how important good oral hygiene is!

Changes to bowel habits

Changes to bowel habits in people approaching the end of life can have a huge effect on quality of life, leading to pain, discomfort, anxiety and possible loss of dignity. This can influence their life to the extent that people become preoccupied with bowel function further affecting their quality of life. Common changes in bowel habit can be at either extreme – constipation or diarrhoea. Of the two, constipation tends to be the more common. For some people they may alternate between the two, leaving them unsure of which may affect them and when.

Constipation

Constipation is the infrequent passing of hard stools. 'Infrequent' can be different for different people – for some people infrequent might mean opening their bowels every other day when they are used to opening their bowels every day. For others, infrequent might mean once a week; for others, once a week might be frequent enough.

Constipation can be an issue for anyone and eating more fibre as part of a balanced diet, drinking more and exercising should always be recommended. For people approaching the end of life, these suggestions can be more difficult to achieve, for example, having an adequate, balanced diet and drinking plenty of fluids. This can be a struggle for those at the end of their life when they may be experiencing a reduced or absent appetite and are unable to tolerate a normal diet and large quantities of fluid. Often the medications given to relieve other symptoms may worsen constipation. An example is the use of pain medication. Constipation may also add to other symptoms; it may make the person feel bloated, or cause discomfort and pain; they may complain of nausea or even vomit as a result.

Think about a person you have cared for who felt constipated. What was their normal pattern of bowel motions? Would they normally expect to pass a motion every day, every other day, once a week? What is usual for them? How do they feel if their usual pattern changes? Ask if this is a common problem and, if so, what has helped in the past? Finding out the answers to these questions may help to guide you about what to advise.

Once you have fully assessed the person, it may be possible to offer some advice. Encourage the person to drink as much as they are able and assist them if they need help to do so.

Talk to them about their usual diet and discuss the benefits of a diet that is high in fibre, wholemeal bread or wholewheat pasta or rice, fruit and vegetables for example. The benefits of this should be balanced against the person's ability to tolerate this.

Movement may help, for some it may be a gentle walk, for others this may be simple exercises in bed, or gently rubbing the abdomen. Constipation can be a lifelong problem for some people – ask what they have found useful in the past. Some people may rely on taking 'natural remedies' such as prunes, dried fruit, prune or fruit juices, nuts and pulses, dark chocolate or syrup of figs. This list is not exhaustive and individual to the person who may have their own ideas about remedies.

Going to the toilet is a very private thing and it is important to ensure as much privacy as possible. This can be difficult because of the situations in which we sometimes care for people. We need to balance the need for a toilet or commode to be in a private place while close at hand. Thought needs to go into how to best manage this, especially if the person is fatigued. Wheeling them to the bathroom could be a solution. Being aware of the usual position when sitting on the toilet could be useful; for example, opening bowels can be easier if knees are higher than hips, so placing the feet on a step will raise knees and may help.

If people continue to have problems opening their bowels, then it may be necessary to use laxatives. Laxatives are medicines that help either to soften the stool or to stimulate the bowel. Some will be combination of both. There are many different laxatives available – some of them are available over the counter at the chemist, while others need to be prescribed. If the problem is more persistent or causing other symptoms, or may be related to other medicines, the GP may need to be asked to review the situation.

Jenny's need for privacy

Jenny is now bed-bound. Her bed is in the dining room and her husband and daughter have made her new bedroom very pleasant and comfortable. Jenny can, with help, move from the bed to the commode. She accepts that the commode is necessary, but it is a constant reminder of her declining health and she hates it. Her daughter comes up with the simple solution that a throw and cushions will disguise the commode when not in use. It has become Jenny's granddaughter's favourite place to sit.

Diarrhoea

Diarrhoea is generally defined as passing stools that are loose in consistency and more frequent than three times daily. However, diarrhoea can be defined differently by different people and may or may not be a problem to them. Again, assessing the person may help determine the cause of the problem and how much impact it is having on the person's quality of life. This is particularly important as treatment is very different depending on the cause of the diarrhoea.

Sometimes severe constipation can lead to the passing of a liquid stool – this liquid leaks past the hard stool. In this situation the person may complain of diarrhoea when in fact they need medication to relieve the hard stool in their bowel. This stool may be referred to as 'overflow' and will need either a nurse or GP to assess and treat. Treatment may be a combination of different measures including the use of suppositories (a softening agent inserted into the back passage to lubricate) and laxatives.

However, diarrhoea can be due to other causes and so may be short lasting – just because someone is considered to be in the last part of their lives, they may still experience common and typical reasons for loose stools, for example, upset stomach, food poisoning, and viruses, etc. In this circumstance, it is advised:

- to encourage the person to drink as much as possible to replace fluid lost with the diarrhoea, this could include rehydration sachets available over the counter or on prescription;
- to encourage small frequent meals which are easy to digest;
- to think about using a barrier cream to soothe or prevent any soreness around the anus;
- to seek advice from the GP if diarrhoea is persistent. The GP may be able to identify a cause and consider medications to slow down the loose stools.

The GP will also be aware of the person's medical history and so could advise whether any changes to the bowel habits may be related to this and if so require specific management.

Poor appetite

When someone is feeling less well, their appetite is often reduced. Appetite may also be affected by many other symptoms, for example, nausea and vomiting, changes to bowel habits, pain, memory problems and shortness of breath. Each of these is covered elsewhere in this chapter. In addition, as disease progresses, general fatigue and, for some, the slowing down of food absorption can also affect appetite. Food should not be forced, it should be encouraged. Simple measures may include attractively presented small meals and having snacks readily at hand. Food that is easy to swallow and digest, such as ice cream, jelly, or high fat yogurts, is often easier to eat.

Supplement drinks and puddings (such as Fortisips, Fortipuds, Complan, Build-ups, etc.) can be used as replacement meals. Check that the person enjoys these – there is nothing worse than being offered something that is not agreeable! The old adage 'a bit of what you fancy does you good' fits here. Having a stock of readily available treats, or having a stock of possible treats easily at hand, can be an effective means of increasing calorie intake. Adding cream to soups, cheese to mashed potato, ice-cream to supplement drinks means that even though a small amount is eaten, additional sustenance is ingested. Check, though, that the person feels they can cope with richer foods.

It may be possible to stimulate appetite with medication, such as low dose steroids. The person's GP would need to prescribe the steroids and monitor the effectiveness and use of this medication. A pre-dinner sherry or a glass of wine with lunch can also act as an appetite stimulant and can help the person enjoy the experience of eating, making it more social than functional. If alcohol is to be offered, it is important to check that this can be taken with any medication that is prescribed.

Food is an important part of life and a social event in itself, so eating alone can be isolating for a significant number of people. Food sustains but also has a strong community element – think of all the celebratory meals for weddings, birthdays or meals for religious occasions such as Christmas, Diwali or the Jewish celebration of Hanukah. Loss of appetite can be very upsetting for the person's family. They may take it personally and perceive lack of appetite as 'giving up', not only on food, but on life and possibly even themselves. Part of caring can be providing food and so family members can feel that they are letting someone down by not encouraging this.

Families often want to try and feed their relatives, believing that nutrition is essential. This can be distressing to people who are nearing the end of life, who don't feel that they want to eat or can't tolerate large amounts of food. It can be an additional pressure for the person and those who care for them. Although the suggested strategies listed above may be helpful, even these may create a degree of distress for the people involved. Because of this, it is important that the person you are caring for and their families are able to talk about any issues regarding food. Families may need your help to understand that, as someone becomes more unwell, they do not necessarily need as much food and that this may not concern the individual themselves.

Maria's appetite and her family

Food has always been an important part of Maria's life. She has only recently retired from the family's restaurant. She has always shown her love for her husband and children by cooking for them, but since she has become less well, she has stopped cooking and her breathlessness means she is eating less and less. Her daughters have always been telling her she should be watching her weight but now it is them that are slipping double cream into her tomato soup and extra butter into the mashed potatoes! Maria has never been much of a drinker but the small sherry the GP suggested before meals seems to help her appetite a little.

Poor mobility and loss of independence

As a person's illness progresses, it may affect their ability to move about and carry out activities in their daily life – this can be the usual pattern of change with their illness. However, if there are any sudden and unexpected changes in mobility, then there should be an urgent review by the person's doctor or nurse. Various treatments such as radiotherapy, chemotherapy and medications can affect a person's mobility, as well as disease progression, general weakness, or having an infection.

If the person is less mobile, be aware that there is an increased risk of developing pressure sores. These sores are related to the difficulty in changing position, so encouraging or helping the person to move regularly may help prevent any problems. Check areas exposed to pressure such as the bottom, ears, and the heels for redness or soreness – if you notice any changes in the skin, it may be necessary to report this to the doctor or nurse just in case they can suggest a solution such as a barrier cream or equipment which reduces the pressure of sitting or lying. It may be that a specialist pressure-relieving cushion or mattress is required.

Find out what equipment you have available where you work. Do you have specialist pressure-relieving cushions and mattresses? If not, where can you get hold of them? Who would be able to advise you?

The realisation that they need help can be upsetting for a person and many people struggle to ask for it. It is important that we acknowledge this and offer the opportunity for the person to be able to talk about their feelings around this. Advice and support are available from other professionals, for example, a physiotherapist who can assess mobility and who, if appropriate, may be able to suggest exercises to improve or maintain a person's mobility. They may provide an appropriate walking aid and work closely with an occupational therapist to help the person to remain as independent as possible. A physiotherapist and occupational therapist can carry out comprehensive assessments of a person's mobility and activities of daily living. They will aim to minimise the risk of falls and carer injury. They can advise on techniques, for example, sit rather than stand and dress the weaker area first. An occupational therapist can arrange for the provision of equipment designed to ensure the person remains as independent as possible for as long as possible, without exacerbating or worsening their symptoms.

For some people approaching the end of their life, a slow deterioration in their mobility and independence is normal and your role is simply to support them to adjust and cope with the deterioration in their condition.

Some other questions that should be considered include:

- Is the person unsteady on their feet?
- Does someone need to be with them while they are moving about?

- Has the person fallen or do they stumble or complain of difficulty with balance?
- Is it more difficult for the person to manage stairs?
- Does the person struggle to get up from a sitting position?
- Does the person struggle to get comfortable in bed or move from a lying to sitting position when getting out of bed?
- Can the person get in and out of their home or are there difficulties with access?
- Are washing and dressing becoming more difficult?
- Can the person get in and out of the bath/shower?
- Would any additional grab rails or equipment be helpful? (For example, raising the height of a chair or sofa, therefore making it easier to get up.)
- Does the person struggle with domestic tasks such as meal preparation and housework/laundry?

It can be helpful to have a look around the person's home or environment and see if there is anything straightforward which can be done to help, for instance:

- moving rugs or anything else which could be a potential trip hazard;
- moving any clutter which might get in the way of a walking aid;
- ensuring there are walking aids available both upstairs and downstairs;
- helping people 'furniture walk', having various handholds around the house, while you observe them walking around and checking that the handholds they use are secure. Could furniture be moved around to make it safer?
- cutlery with larger handles can be helpful or adapt existing cutlery with foam tubing. Non-slip mats can be helpful under plates.
- could food be ordered online rather than having to visit the supermarket?
- keeping commonly used items within easy reach to avoid bending and stretching;
- buying aids to daily living activities available online or at disability equipment stores.

So far, this chapter has highlighted some of the symptoms that a person may experience. These may vary in severity and may come and go, but if not managed effectively can have a dramatic effect on the quality of life for the person experiencing it. There are multiple ways in which symptoms can be managed without the use of drugs. For some people, medication will be necessary and the next section of the chapter will focus on some of the most common drugs that may be used.

The use of medication to manage symptoms

How is medication given?

Giving medication via the mouth is always the first route of choice. For the people that we care for, this is not always possible. For example, if someone is experiencing nausea or vomiting, they will not be able to take tablets; it is entirely possible that they won't want to take tablets. For some people, as they become increasingly unwell, swallowing may become difficult. Some of the people that we care for have dementia and may be reluctant to have anything in their mouth. For people in these diffferent situations, alternative means of medication will need to be found.

Routes of administration of medication

- *Oral* – tablets, lozenges or liquids. Check the way that the tablet is to be given – swallowed whole, placed under the tongue (sub-lingual), put between the gum and the cheek (buccal). Other tablets may require disolving in water. Many medications are also avilable in liquid form.
- *Suppositories* – some pain medications can be given in the form of suppositories in the back passage. To administer in this way may require some additional training and for some people will be unacceptable on a regular basis.
- *Patches* – strong pain-relieving and anti-sickness drugs can be given by using a medication patch (often referred to as a transdermal patch) that is stuck onto the skin. The patch is replaced regularly – this may be every three to four days, daily or weekly depending on the type of drug and the prescription. They have the advantage that medications can be given with minimal disruption to the person, offering a constant dose of medication. It is important to remember that these are still powerful drugs and should be dispensed according to the prescription given.
- *Injections* – Some people may require reqular injections to replace deficiencies such as iron. These are usually given

monthly. Medications for pain and nausea can also be given via injection. These are usually administered into the subcutaneous tissue using a short needle.

● *Continuous infusion via a pump* – if the person is unable to take medication by mouth, or is requiring frequent injections to help manage their symptoms, it may be necessary to give these freqent medications using a **syringe pump** over 24 hours. This method, discussed in more detail at the end of the chapter, can be helpful in end of life care as medication can be given continually so that the levels remain constant and it avoids regular injections, which can be painful and difficult to administer regularly.

Managing pain with medication

For some people, medication will not be necessary, for others it may be the only thing that will help, but for most a combination of the techniques already described, including medication, will be most helpful. A key principle of effective pain medication can be summed up in Figure 5.1: medication given (1) by mouth; (2) by clock; (3) by ladder.

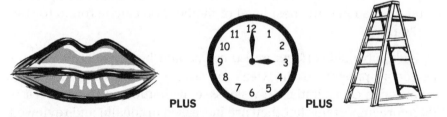

PLUS   **PLUS**

Figure 5.1 Effective pain medication methods

Getting the right medication to manage a specific pain can be challenging. If pain medication is necessary for chronic ongoing pain, medication (analgesics) should be given regularly, not just when the pain is at its worse. Ideally this should be given by the *mouth*: medications given orally can be better tolerated and less distressing for the person to take than, for example, frequent injections or suppositories. The medication should be given by the *clock*: given at regular intervals throughout the day so there is a constant level within the bloodstream. If medicines were taken as needed, there may be long gaps in between doses and this might result in episodes of pain once the medications' effect has worn off. Finally, by the *ladder*: this is the gradual increasing of the strength of painkilling medications, dependent on need.

Pain medication can be divided into three groups:

- weak
- moderate
- strong

The person is usually started on a weak painkiller. This can be very effective for a number of different types of pain. They may be used in combination with other drugs such as anti-inflammatories. If this does not reduce the pain, then the next step of the ladder is to give the person moderate painkillers, often referred to as 'weak opioids'. **Opioids** are morphine-derived drugs. Weak opioids commonly include codeine-based drugs and can be given with paracetamol; often codeine can be available in tablets combined with paracetamol, for example, co-codamol. If the pain is persistent and severe, and not helped by the previous drugs described in the earlier two steps, then they may step up to a strong opioid-based painkiller. Morphine is an example of a commonly used strong opioid, but you may also come across oxycodone, buprenorphine or fentanyl. The reason that this stepped approach is taken is so that the best level of medication can be found for the person.

Opioids have side-effects and these should be considered when a person is prescribed the weak or strong medicines. Commonly, opioids can cause initial drowsiness, constipation and nausea – it is therefore important that they are increased gradually and reviewed regularly. Some of the techniques given earlier in the chapter may be useful in helping to manage these side-effects.

Jenny's painkillers

Jenny finds it increasingly difficult to get comfortable and feels that as her pain increases, she can no longer cope with it. Jenny initially had occasional pain and so she would take paracetamol every now and again when it got too much for her. The GP, Dr Rowland, sees Jenny at his surgery because of her increasing pain. He suggests taking the paracetamol regularly throughout the day, taking the maximum, for Jenny that is two tablets every 6 hours, but no more than eight tablets in every

24-hour period. This works for a few months, but gradually Jenny begins to recognise that the pain is bothering her again. Dr Rowland suggests stepping up to the moderate painkiller, co-codamol. She stops the paracetamol and takes regular co-codamol tablets. She complains again that her pain has returned. Dr Rowland recommends morphine – a low dose at first but she can have more if she needs it. Jenny's husband Stephen hates to see her in pain but is very concerned about her starting morphine as he says, 'she will become addicted'.

Dr Rowland sits with Stephen (and Jenny) and calmly explains that as it is being given to control pain rather than for 'recreational' purposes, it is not addictive. It is likely that the morphine will cause constipation and that some people can initially feel sick and a bit sleepy when they first start it. The GP checks that Jenny has both an anti-sickness medication and something in case of constipation.

Stephen is very relieved and Jenny starts on the liquid morphine, taking some every four hours. She can also have an extra 'break-through' dose if she needs it in between her regular doses.

Other medications to control pain

Other medications may also help control pain and discomfort, though they are not painkillers. These are described as **adjuvant**, meaning medications that work in combination with others. For example, if a person gets heartburn, it may help if they receive antacid medications, sit upright when eating, avoid foods that worsen the heartburn, or eat small and frequent meals.

If you are unsure about medications being given, think about how you might find some more advice. Who else may be involved in their care? See **Chapter 3** for more information about those who may be involved in supporting the person's care needs.

We would aim to provide medication regularly, by mouth, but in some cases this is not possible. This could be related to other symptoms, for example, if a person was feeling sick or being sick.

The use of anti-sickness medication

Many of the suggestions given earlier in the chapter will help with the unpleasant feeling of nausea and vomiting. As well as these important measures, there are also different anti-sickness medications (anti-emetics) which may offer some relief. Some anti-sickness medications can also be purchased over the counter from a chemist or pharmacy. The person you are caring for may well have tried some of these purchased medicines and so it is important to ask if this is the case and if they have been useful. Some of these medicines would need to be prescribed by a doctor. Assessing the cause, where possible, will determine the treatment required, as the different anti-sickness medications work in different ways for different causes.

Ideally, just like pain management, it is better to offer medicines by mouth. However, if nausea and vomiting are severe and persistent, and a person is unable to tolerate anything by mouth, they may require drugs given by either injection or via a syringe pump, which will need the involvement of the person's GP and nurse. This can often improve symptoms to the extent that people will be able to start taking diet, fluids and potentially medication by mouth and therefore improve their experiences and quality of life.

Medications for breathlessness

There may be certain prescribed medications that may help relieve the sensation of breathlessness. Small doses of opioid-based medications, for example, morphine, can decrease the sensation of breathlessness, making breathing seem easier. Medications used to treat anxiety can also be helpful, particularly when the person is feeling anxious as a result of their worsening sensation of breathlessness.

Oxygen, inhalers and nebulisers

Oxygen may not be helpful for all people experiencing breathlessness, but for some it is necessary and can bring comfort. Home oxygen and portable oxygen are available. Many people receiving oxygen therapy in these situations say that the greatest benefit is the feeling of air movement across the face, so it worth thinking about whether there are other ways that this could be achieved. Depending on the cause of the breathlessness, **nebulisers** and inhalers can help open up the airway, to relieve the sensation of shortness of breath – again, for some, this is beneficial but may not benefit all. For this reason, these should only be used as prescribed.

The use of syringe pumps at the end of life

As we have seen in this chapter, the majority of care at the end of life does not involve complex medication regimes. Sometimes, however, with guidance, specific drugs may be appropriate to ensure the person's maximum comfort. As the person becomes increasingly drowsy and their swallowing reflex less strong, routes other than by mouth need to be explored. Medication can be administered via suppositories into the rectum, which while effective can be uncomfortable and for some unacceptable. Alternatively medication can be administered via injection. This can be a one-off dose known as a 'stat' or as required (often referred to as PRN). If, however, the medication is required more regularly, then a pump may be set up. This is a small lightweight battery-operated pump. A short needle is placed under the skin and secured with a light dressing. As the needle is placed in subcutaneous tissue, the ideal places for insertion are the more 'plump' areas such as the top of the arm, stomach or top of the thigh. For people who are confused, the shoulder can be the least disruptive. There is a clear LCD display which provides information such as how long until the pump needs changing or if the battery level is low. The pump is attached to the person with a length of tubing, which can be discreetly placed under a pillow.

The McKinley T34 syringe pump is one of the most popular and has been adopted as the pump of choice by the NHS (Figure 5.2). Pumps have the advantage over 'stat' injections in that the person is injected less frequently (each pump will last for 24 hours). Another major advantage is that it is possible to get constant drug levels rapidly. In this chapter we have mentioned a combination of drugs that can be helpful at the end of life. Multiple drugs can be given in the same syringe, so one syringe in a pump could give a constant dose of pain relief, medication to reduce chesty secretions, anti-sickness and something to help the person feel calmer and settled. The use of a syringe pump should be seen as the exception rather than the norm for many of the people that we are caring for. Its use is supported by either the district nurse, GP or by the palliative care or hospice team, depending on where the person is being cared. Day-to-day management of the pump could be by registered nurses in a nursing home, the district nurses in a residential care home or a carer in someone's own home (who usually organises their own training).

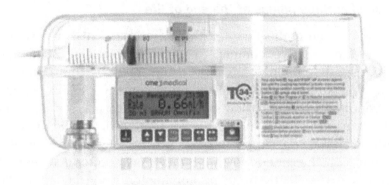

Figure 5.2 The McKinley T34 syringe pump
Source: Permission courtesy of the manufacturer.

This chapter has considered some of the symptoms a person may experience at the end of their life. These can vary in severity and can be frightening for the person, but also alarming to those caring for them. This chapter has highlighted the simple things that can make a difference.

**Helping people manage the common physical symptoms at the end of life:
things to remember**

- Consider the commonly experienced symptoms discussed in this chapter. How do you check if someone is experiencing any symptoms?
- Assess the person if they are experiencing a symptom. What do you see, what do they tell you, how are they feeling, is there a change in the person?
- Monitor and record changes in the person's condition, however small.
- Consider *all* actions to relieve the symptom. Some of these you can do, others you may need to refer to a healthcare professional or specialist.

- If the symptom persists, question whether there is anything that you have missed. What would you do next? Where could you get more information about how to help? Who else could advise or support the person, yourself and their family?
- Keep in mind that the person is the expert in what they are experiencing!

 Chapter 6 will focus on some of the non-physical symptoms that a person may experience which can be as equally distressing as their physical counterparts.

What are the common non-physical symptoms and concerns at the end of life and how can we help?

Christine Linley, Belinda Hitchens and Karen Cook

Non-physical symptoms can be as significant as those physical symptoms discussed previously. This chapter will:

- identify the common non-physical symptoms experienced as the end of life approaches;
- focus on how you might recognise these in the person you are caring for;
- offer suggestions to help you support the person experiencing these symptoms and how you can help manage them.

A person can experience a range of physical symptoms and in Chapter 5 we learnt that there are a number of things that we can do to help. This chapter will focus on some of the other symptoms that a person may experience as they approach the end of their life and will focus on those with a non-physical or a psychological element. The symptoms to be considered are:

- tiredness and fatigue;
- difficulty sleeping;
- alterations in mood;
- confusion;
- anxiety;
- sexual issues.

Tiredness and fatigue

Tiredness and fatigue can be distressing symptoms that can seriously affect a person's quality of life. They can occur as a result of the underlying disease, their general condition or sometimes as a side-effect of treatments and medications such as chemotherapy or radiotherapy. It is important to note that tiredness and fatigue are not the same. Tiredness is a sensation that many of us feel after a busy day or if we have had a disturbed night's sleep, but fatigue is different to just feeling tired. It can be overwhelming and get in the way of being able to carry out everyday activities. Often the feeling of fatigue is not relieved by sleep or a rest. For some people, fatigue can affect their ability to function physically, socially, psychologically, often affecting their ability to think through issues (their cognition). We will briefly look at these four areas and the impact of fatigue on each.

Fatigue can affect a person *physically*; insomnia (where they struggle to sleep) or, the opposite, hypersomnia (wanting to sleep all the time) can be a problem. Some people can sleep, but they may find that the experience of sleep isn't refreshing and this can lead to a loss of strength and energy with associated weakness, limb heaviness and feeling exhausted after any activity, even if this activity is small. This weakness can make them at an increased risk of falling; they may also find that their appetite changes and reduces.

Socially, fatigue can also cause loss of independence and therefore a change in the person's role in life, for example, they may be unable to work and unable to take on their normal responsibilities within their family. Fatigue can lead to the person becoming socially withdrawn due to feeling unable to engage in relationships.

From a *psychological* point of view, the person can experience feelings of guilt associated with their reduced activity levels; they can feel low in mood and suffer from increased anxiety; the person can feel very 'up and down' and might be more irritable.

The ability to think through and process (a person's *cognition*) may be affected. The person's ability to concentrate may be impaired, making it difficult to read, watch TV or even take part in a conversation. They may struggle to remember things because they are so exhausted.

Maria feeling fatigued

Maria has always been at the heart of her large family. She is becoming more and more fatigued and struggling to carry out the most simple of tasks – even writing a shopping list is exhausting and she keeps forgetting even the simple things. Her daughter, Nancy, is in charge now. She does the shopping but never manages to get it quite right, let alone cook to Maria's exacting standards. Maria feels angry but also guilty – this was her job, but she just can't muster the energy to carry it out. Her family have encouraged her to rest but 'cat naps' didn't make any difference. It all feels too much, she becomes upset and cries that she just wanted to be 'back to normal'. Nancy is becoming increasingly irritated with her mum; frustrated that she can never get it right and her mum won't let her or her family help.

Think about Maria, what do you think may help her manage her fatigue? How would you reassure her family about how Maria is feeling?

The feeling of tiredness and fatigue can be overwhelming and difficult to manage. The 'Five Ps' can be a useful way of remembering things that may help:

1. *Plan.* Think about what tasks need to be done and whether they can be broken down into more manageable steps. It can be helpful to keep a diary of when fatigue is at its worst and plan to perform more effortful tasks when they have the most energy, for example, mornings may be better, evenings may be worse. Think about the week – have they got appointments or activities that are important? – if so, think about having a rest day before and after in order to prepare and recover.
2. *Prioritise* what has to be done and what is important to the person – leave what can be left to another day. Ask for help, for example, if it is important for the people to wash themselves, could they get some support with dressing?
3. *Pacing* and taking regular rests. Try not to do everything all in one go. Have chairs around the house so it is easy to sit and rest when required. Break tasks down into smaller parts and rest in between.
4. *Positioning.* For example, can the person sit rather than stand to perform certain tasks? Install grab rails to assist with showering/bathing, mobility and transferring from bed to chair, an occupational therapist may be able to help with this.
5. *Permission.* Encourage the person to give themselves a rest if that is what they feel they need to do. It may also be important

to ensure that carers, family and friends are aware of how fatigue associated with illness can have a huge impact on the person's daily life – that it isn't just being tired.

Discovering ways of conserving energy is important. This can be practical things such as avoiding unnecessary journeys up or down the stairs and ensuring furniture is at the correct height. It can also be helpful to ensure that items are at the correct height in cupboards to avoid unnecessary bending and reaching.

Even though the person may not feel like it, some light exercise can be helpful in managing fatigue and make sleep or rest more effective. Trying to build some exercise into the person's daily routine can be helpful. If exercise is impossible, try to encourage the person to remain as active as they can within their daily routine and ability.

Some people find a fatigue diary useful – writing down when they experience fatigue. Ask the person to complete a fatigue diary and then look at it together and identify any times when their energy 'leaks'. Then together think about how they could adapt either by a change of routine or maybe through using a piece of equipment.

Difficulty sleeping

Sleep can be an issue for someone who is fatigued; it also can, however, be an issue for other people facing a serious illness and uncertain future. This could be because their symptoms are not adequately controlled, because they are napping more and more in the day, or because they are worried or upset. Whatever is causing difficulty in sleeping, it is important to pay attention to 'good sleep hygiene', which is a bedtime routine that supports settling and falling off to sleep. This can include some of the following ideas:

- Try to go to bed at a regular time and get up at a regular time each day.
- Avoid caffeine and alcohol before bed; maybe try a milky drink, or reading beforehand.
- Practise a relaxation exercise before going to sleep.
- Ensure that the room is the right temperature; ideally, limit daytime naps to 45 minutes.
- Avoid using mobile phones, computers or watching TV immediately before going to sleep.

Change in mood

When a person is unwell and having to come to terms with the end of their life it can of course affect their mood and how they feel about themselves. The loss of independence and needing to depend on others can be frustrating and depressing. Pain and fatigue can also make a person feel depressed. The person might also feel anxious. There are symptoms which can occur at the end of life which can cause feelings of anxiety and even panic, such as breathlessness. There are difficult decisions to be made such as deciding on the person's preferred place of care or death, along with tasks such as trying to ensure that their affairs are in order. All of this can cause the person to feel overwhelmed.

How could you help the person who seems depressed or low in mood?

Helping someone who is low in mood can be hard as their feeling of depression may mean that they can see no positives. In **Chapter 4** we discussed how important talking can be. Allow the person to talk about how they feel if that is what they want to do. We may need to pick up on cues. They may say that they are 'OK' but you can see from the way they are looking or sitting that this may not be the case. You can learn a lot from the simple question: 'Are you sure you are OK?' Remember that your words or advice may not bring about a change in the person's situation, but listening and allowing the person to express their feelings may ease their distress. Sometimes, a person would prefer to talk about feelings with someone other than those close to them for fear of hurting them. It is not uncommon for someone to express the fact that they are ready to die, but it can be hard for those close to them to hear.

It can be worth asking if there is anything in particular that is worrying them. It may be that a simple solution can be found that may help raise their mood. Distraction can be effective but needs to be used once the cause of the low mood is identified. Without this, distraction can help the carer but not the person who is cared for, it can feel like the cause of the low mood is being swept aside. Distraction can, however, be helpful in many situations. It may be that they have visitors whom they would enjoy seeing, or perhaps going somewhere else, or just doing something different, would have a positive influence. Anti-depressants can be helpful but should be given under the direction of a medical practitioner. These can sometimes lift a person's mood enough to enable them to manage to express themselves more easily and get on with life.

Ways to help when a person is feeling anxious

Remain calm and reassure the person, tell them that you will do what you can to help, perhaps offer to stay with them. Encourage the person to slow their breathing. When anxious or panicking, our breathing rate quickens and this is responsible for many of the uncomfortable symptoms associated with anxiety and panic attacks. Slowing the breathing rate significantly reduces the physical symptoms associated with anxiety. It can be helpful to count when breathing in and out, making the out-breath last longer than the in-breath, for example, breathing in to the count of 3 and out to the count of 5. This can be practised regularly throughout the day. Try to encourage the person to breathe from lower down in their lungs, this is achieved when the person's stomach rises and falls during breathing. If a person's shoulders are rising and falling as they breathe, this is a sign that they are breathing shallowly. It may also be helpful to involve a carer or significant other so they can become aware of the signs that anxiety levels are rising and prompt them to use coping strategies.

- Listening to some relaxing music can be helpful.
- Practising relaxation exercises daily can be helpful in reducing the background level of anxiety a person experiences. A healthcare professional, such as an occupational therapist can advise you on these. Relaxation CDs can also easily be purchased online.
- Distracting the person from their anxious thoughts can also help.
- Identify if there is something that triggers the feelings of anxiety. Talking about their feelings can be helpful. Depending on your place of work, you may have access to an occupational therapist, psychologist, a complementary therapist, a hypnotherapist, art or music therapist.
- If the anxiety is the result of breathlessness, there are strategies which can be helpful, see section on breathlessness in **Chapter 5**.

Find out what other services are available in your local area to support people who are struggling to manage how they feel. Find out what these services can offer and how to contact them.

Confusion and changes in ability to understand and reason

Confusion can be a common problem at the end of life and very distressing for the person experiencing it, as well as their family and carers. There may be many reasons why their ability to understand and reason could be affected, for example, this can be due to underlying disease process, infection, depression, medication side-effects, pain or a chemical imbalance such as abnormally high levels of calcium in the blood. All of these are potentially reversible. The person may have already had a condition which impairs their ability to understand and reason such as dementia.

How can we help a person who is confused?

Regardless of the cause, the same principles apply. Remain calm and try not to correct or argue with the person. This can be hard but remember it is not necessary to always tell the person that they are wrong about something. Does it really matter? When a person's memory fails, they are living in a world where they are constantly being told they are wrong, 'No, it's not Monday, it's Tuesday', 'No, that was 10 years ago not 2 years ago.' It can be important to gently remind the person of some things, but there may be times when it is best to 'let it go'. If the person has difficulty remembering names, encourage them to use a person's name as much as possible during conversation. Encourage the person to have a routine, to be as organised as possible. **Dossette boxes** can assist with taking medication correctly. Pharmacies can deliver these with the medication arranged in blister packs for the times of the day and days of the week. This is particularly helpful for checking whether a person is taking their medication correctly. Fatigue and sleep diaries can be helpful, as can a regular diary or calendar, which can help someone who is confused, if they remember to look at it. This strategy will be more successful for someone who has always been in the habit of using a diary. Keeping a pocket notebook and pen can also be useful, so the person is always able to write things down.

If a person is confused and at home, safety issues with appliances, particularly gas appliances, will need to be considered. Check if there is an automatic safety cut-off valve ensuring the gas cuts off if not lit. Isolation switches can be fitted to gas appliances, meaning that the appliance can be operated by a carer but not by the person who is confused. Ensure that smoke alarms are fitted and regularly checked. There are special devices that can be inserted into sinks/basins, which alert you to temperature and cut off water supply prior to overflowing. An occupational therapist will be able to provide advice.

Some people take great pleasure from going out and, if this is case, it is advisable that they have their name and address with them if they are still able to go out on their own and there is a risk of them getting lost. Talisman bracelets can be purchased online or from good pharmacies. These can have details of a person's medical condition and contact details for a relative in case of emergency. Alternatively, the person could just have a card with these details in their wallet/purse or in the pocket of their coat. If eating and drinking become an issue, then it may be helpful to try to differentiate items, for example, have plain white plates on a coloured background with coloured bands around the cutlery. Sometimes, when someone needs to be transferred to an unfamiliar environment, for example, into hospital or a hospice, it can be helpful to ensure that they have some familiar things around them, such as pictures, objects, own bedding or pillow – and, if possible, it helps to get an idea about usual rou-

tines, likes and dislikes and trying to incorporate them as much as practically possible. More information on confusion at the end of life can be found in **Chapter 9**.

How can we tell if someone is struggling with their mood?

How would we recognise that a person's mood and the way they are feeling has changed? Are they withdrawn; not wanting to meet with friends? Do they struggle to sleep at night and is it difficult for them to talk openly about their worries and concerns? Or do they continuously verbalise their worries; do they appear anxious and does this prevent them from carrying out their own personal care? What about someone who is struggling to understand or accept their changing situation?

Depression and anxiety can be present and can be recognised by different signs and symptoms:

- low mood, feelings of hopelessness and sadness, sometimes feeling worse at a particular time of the day, commonly in the morning or overnight;
- feelings of guilt;
- the inability to take pleasure in anything;
- crying;
- difficulties with attention and concentration so that even reading or watching TV becomes impossible;
- poor appetite;
- changes in sleep pattern, for example, difficulty sleeping;
- lack of motivation;
- feelings of being unable to cope and wanting to end their life;
- anxiety/panic (this can cause many further symptoms such as giddiness, palpitations, chest tightness, sweating, trembling, a dry mouth, shortness of breath or a choking sensation, changes in hearing and vision, tingling in the hands and feet, stomach discomfort). A panic attack can be a very frightening experience and can happen suddenly and without apparent cause.

Think about the signs listed above. How would you find out if the person was experiencing any of these? Think about how you would ask if they were feeling any of these difficulties.

Sexual issues

Sexuality and sexual issues do not stop being important because a person is dying. It can be a significant issue, but one that we often find difficult to discuss with the people we care for and therefore can be ignored or minimised. It can feel embarrassing and we can question how appropriate it is to discuss it, but it can be very significant to the person, so, despite being a challenge, it should not be avoided. While older people may express intimacy in a different way than when they were younger, it would be wrong to believe that age necessarily stops the expression of sexual desire. A person's sexuality is not just about sexual activity but about much more. It includes gender roles, identity and how a person likes to express and experience intimacy. Sexual problems are common and may be due to a number or reasons. They may be as a direct result of illness, treatment, or related to anxiety, depression or mood change. When someone is dying, they will often have a different view of their body – their body image is altered – and this can lead to low self-esteem. Sexual issues may seem difficult to discuss and seem to be best avoided but there are simple things that we can do to help.

One way that we can help is to make the person feel special – it may be helping them to wash their hair, dressing for a specific occasion or offering a woman a manicure. A man may have always been clean-shaven and this is an important part of his daily ritual. A woman may express the need to wear make-up – 'no one should ever see me without it'. It can be important to discover whether the person has a specific perfume/aftershave they like to use. These may seem simple daily care tasks, but if done with sensitivity and responsiveness, they can make a big difference to how they feel about themselves. Another simple thing we can do is to ensure that the person has privacy, it may be that at times they want to be on their own or feel that they want uninterrupted time with someone important to them. When someone is unwell, this can be difficult to achieve, there may be lots of people 'coming and going' or they may be cared for in an area that lacks privacy, for example, in a shared bedroom, somewhere away from their own home or in a living room. Sensitive and, at times, creative solutions will need to be found.

It is important to know who is important to the person that we are caring for. There can be complicated dynamics – for example, someone who is married but had a mistress for many years, or someone in a same-sex relationship that others have found hard to accept.

Think about how you might feel if you were unable to have some privacy. How might you be able to make this possible for the people in your care? Think about how you could help those you are caring for to experience some time alone with their partner.

Jenny being with Stephen

Jenny accepts that she is finding it harder to get upstairs, spending more time in bed. The district nurse says she will get a hospital/profiling bed with an air loss mattress to prevent Jenny from getting a sore bottom from lying in the same position; they can change the dining room into a bedroom. This district nurse is satisfied that she has found a solution. Jenny, however, is distraught; 'I just want to sleep next to Stephen; I don't want to be on my own without him,' she says. The district nurse explains that it might be risky for Jenny to try to move up and down the stairs, and that she is worried about her skin. Jenny is visibly upset, as is Stephen – they explain that they have had a long and very close marriage and that, at this time in Jenny's life, they understand that time is slipping away and so want to be together as much as they possibly can. They have rarely had a night away from each other. Stephen asks if there is any other solution. The district nurse thinks – one suggestion is that their bed is moved downstairs, into the dining room. The nurse will then order a double overlay pressure-relieving mattress – they will both get the benefit of this pressure-relieving mattress! Stephen sets to organising how to rearrange and move the furniture around.

This simple solution has two benefits. Jenny can be cared for safely in her own home and her and Stephen's wishes to be together have been met.

 Chapter 7 will further discuss Jenny's story and the importance of families and the significant part they have to play at the end of someone's life.

This chapter has focused on some of the non-physical symptoms a person may experience as they approach the end of their life. As has been seen, some of these symptoms may be reversible, others not. Whether the symptoms are physical or non-physical, they should be assessed, monitored and the benefits of any interventions recorded.

As we have seen in this chapter, families play a significant part in the care of a person approaching the end of their life.

What are the common non-physical symptoms at the end of life: things to remember?

- Non-physical symptoms can be as distressing and debilitating as their physical counterparts.
- All symptoms should be considered from the individual's perspective.

- Think about the ways in which you could support and advise the person – what simple steps might help them manage how they are feeling?
- Think about other healthcare professionals who may be able to support the person, identify their concerns and work with you and them to help reach a resolution.

 Chapter 7 will focus on the different roles that people play within families and how we can support their varying needs.

How can we help families?

Liz Reed, Hayley Palfreyman and Sarah Dowd

Most people spend the majority of the last year of their life at home, often with support and care mainly coming from their families. This chapter will focus on:

- the impact on relationships within families when one of its members is dying, from the perspective of a parent, partner and child;
- the importance of communicating with and within families, in particular, how parents can approach difficult conversations with children and the different needs of children at different ages;
- how important it is to have honesty and openness within a family and what can happen if children are not told what is happening;
- activities to help prepare children for the death of a parent or grandparent;
- the importance of a multiprofessional team approach to caring for families.

When someone in a family is dying, it affects everyone. A family can be thrown into chaos as each person thinks about their specific role within the family, for example, their role as parent, partner, child or friend and their relationship with the person who is going to die. Each of them may be experiencing a range of emotions; sadness, anxiety, fear and the burden of feeling responsible for both the person dying and other family members.

We meet families at an important time in their lives. Each person will have their own unique relationship with the dying person. The relationship can be close and loving or can be complicated by difficult events throughout their lives. Sometimes we assume that families are happy and supportive, but in reality for many this is not the case. Knowing that a family member is approaching the end of their life may be an added challenge to a family that is already struggling. So when thinking about how we care for families, we need to ensure we understand, as much as possible, how that family works in order to support them.

Traditionally, families tended to grow up and live in the same town so relatives lived close by and it was easier to support each other. Today, members of one family can live scattered all over the UK or abroad, so caring for each other and the ways we communicate can be very different, for example, Facebook, email, text, Skype, rather than meeting for a cup of tea and a chat.

Each family is unique and will have different dynamics. This chapter will look at how one family is affected by someone dying. We will focus on Jenny Baxter and her family.

Jenny Baxter, her family, and their story

Jenny is a 69-year-old retired administrator and has been married to Stephen for 40 years. They have two adult children; Sarah, who is married, and has two children, Poppy, aged 4 years old and 10-year-old Mark; and Andrew, who is married has one son, Ben, aged 11. Mark lives 200 miles away from his parents. Jenny also has her 91-year-old mother Freda to look after. Freda is frail and lives in a care home in the same town. Jenny has a good relationship with her mother, she visits her three or four times a week in the care home and they have enjoyed day trips together.

Jenny was diagnosed with advanced breast cancer four years ago. She has had four cycles of palliative chemotherapy since her diagnosis. Until recently, she has been fairly well and able to be an active part of her family, which included regular childcare for her daughter's children such as picking them up from school and caring for them in the evenings until Sarah finished work. Jenny and Stephen have had a difficult relationship with their daughter-in-law, which is a source of great sadness to them as they don't see their son and grandson as much as they would like. The relationship with their son and his family is strained.

At her last appointment with her oncologist, he told them there were no further treatments available to her and she should consider 'getting her affairs in order'. This did not come as a surprise to Jenny. She was determined that she should decide what she wanted as she approached the end of her life and the doctor talked to her about advance care planning. Jenny and Stephen then met with their GP, Dr Rowland, and with him they documented together that she wanted to die at home and would not accept treatment such as antibiotics should she develop an infection. The GP said he would ensure others involved in her care were given a copy and Jenny and Stephen had a copy in their home.

 For more information on advance care planning, go to *Chapter 2*.

In the recent months Jenny has deteriorated significantly. Now she is very weak, has lost her appetite, has some pain and is spending most of her time in bed. Her GP has told her and Stephen that she is facing the final phase of her life.

Let's think about how this affects each member of the Baxter family.

Changing roles

The normal balance of relationships within a family will be affected when a member of a family is dying. A natural part of the dying process is that the person can begin to feel a little detached from those around them. Jenny will experience many losses:

- loss of usual roles; wife, mother, daughter, grandparent, friend or caregiver;
- loss of the future; enjoying her retirement with Stephen and seeing her grandchildren grow up;
- loss of her independence, increasingly relying on others to meet her care needs.

Jenny has a number of significant roles within her family. She is close to her mother and daughter and has an active role as caregiver in the lives of two of her grandchildren. She also has a complex relationship with her son's family.

A family that communicates openly with each other may be better able to support those within the family at difficult times. Likewise a family that unites at difficult times may be more likely to be able to support and care for each other. But a diagnosis of life-threatening illness in a family can result in each person being unsure what to say or how to talk to the person who is unwell, or address what is happening, even in the most close-knit family. Usual ways of communicating and behaving can be disrupted, which affects everyone in a family. Talking honestly about dying is hard. No one wants to upset those they love and it may seem easier not to talk about it. But everyone needs to know what is happening in a way they can understand. Everyone needs to be able to have time to adjust and prepare for the end of Jenny's life, whatever their age and relationship with her, they may have things they want to say or things they need to do before Jenny dies. Think about all the people around the dying person, what they are going through practically, emotionally and physically and how you can help.

> Think about a family you have been involved in and all the members of that family. What was their relationship to the dying person? What was their role within the family? How did that family communicate? How do you think the end of life care of their relative might impact on their bereavement? In considering the needs of the family, what did you, or could you have done to support them through the end of life phase and their bereavement?

It is important to acknowledge that each person has a distinct role within the family and they will have specific needs.

The partner

The partner of someone who is dying is facing a stressful and unpredictable future. Most couples have a way that they 'work' together and take on specific roles, one may be the decision-maker or provider, and the other may be more the nurturer. These functions can change when a person is unwell. The sick person will have to relinquish things like cooking; the partner may therefore have to take on unfamiliar tasks. Information and practical and emotional support are key to a partner's ability to fulfil their role, with an ongoing need for information about the present and future, so it is very important to consider the needs of the partner as well as the person who is dying.

The partner's own well being can be at risk as they may have little time to rest and may be less likely to look after themselves when they feel responsible for their relative. Sources of stress for partners can be uncertainty about the future, not enough information about the person who is dying, poor communication between the dying person and the partner, feeling unprepared for their role of carer, taking on additional responsibility within the family, and employment and money worries. Alongside this is the constant anticipation of having to live and cope in the long term without the dying person.

Jenny's husband, Stephen

Stephen fully supports Jenny's advance care plan. He was part of the discussion when they sat with Dr Rowland and drew it up. He understands why she wants to die at home. Stephen, though, is worried he will not be able to look after Jenny as well as he thinks she deserves.

What health and social care roles do you thing would be helpful in supporting Jenny and Stephen to ensure her wishes are respected? How can you support Stephen and prepare him for the end of Jenny's life so that her wishes are honoured?

Taking on other responsibilities the ill person can no longer do can put significant pressure on the caregiver. Tasks that were simple for the dying person may be challenging for others. The burden of care both for the family and the person who is unwell can fall to the partner who may also be balancing caregiving with other responsibilities.

Jenny's and Stephen's roles in the family

Stephen is now providing all practical care for Jenny while thinking about how he will cope without her and the future they looked forward to together. Jenny did everything in the home and now he has to think about cooking, cleaning and looking after himself as well as his wife. He may feel the challenge to be there for all the family both now and in the future without Jenny. He wants to continue to care for his grandchildren but Jenny did most of the practical caring. She loved brushing and braiding her granddaughter Poppy's hair. It was a highlight of Poppy's visits – for both of them. Stephen feels useless; he has never brushed Poppy's hair before and certainly never braided it. His wife is too unwell to tell him how to do it so he searches on the internet and finds a video of how to do it. After some practice he is able to brush and braid the child's hair. But what does this do for a family? Jenny sees her husband slowly taking over the tasks she loved to do, she may feel no longer useful to her grandchild. Stephen feels incompetent but then pleased that he can now take over this role and the grandchild feels both distressed that her grandmother can no longer do this small task for her and guilty that they are coping without her grandmother. Stephen and Poppy are confused as they unwittingly prepare for life after Jenny has died. Stephen feels unprepared as he tries to take over his wife's role, sadness as he sees her get worse and feels guilt that he is beginning to develop the skills he will need when she is gone and, even though he dreads the day, he is preparing for life after her death.

While the focus of your care will be the person who is dying, it is very important that you are able to support the partner too. To do this, think about the following:

- How can you help them to understand about aspects of treatment and care?
- Give them time to talk about their feelings and fears.
- Look at services in your area that offer practical and emotional support to partners and families (they may be social services or charities).
- If the partner is worried about their job and money, seek support from a social worker or Citizens Advice Bureau to see what financial support they can get.

While it is important that the partner is aware of what is happening, think about what you share with them. It is not a good idea for partners to understand more than the dying person about what is happening as this can be a burden to carry and build a barrier between them. Imagine that Jenny is unaware of her prognosis, while Stephen has been told she has just weeks to live. How do you think Stephen would cope with knowing something about his wife that she doesn't? How might it affect how he communicated with her? How would Jenny feel if she found out her husband knew more that she did about her illness and life expectancy?

Adult children

When we think about losing a parent, the focus is most commonly on young children, but losing a parent at any age will be difficult. People say things like: 'Well, he was in his eighties', but to his children he was a dad. The father who celebrated their first words, taught them to ride a bike, walked them down the aisle or bought them their first pint. The parent that watched them grow into adults and have children of their own. Dying in older age is expected and follows the natural course of events, so the needs of adult children can almost be forgotten. Coping with a dying parent and anticipating life without them can be hard, no matter what age they are.

 ### Jenny's children, Sarah and Andrew

Sarah is very close to her mum, Jenny. They enjoy being together and Sarah has always respected her mum's advice and guidance. She also depends on her for support and childcare. She is concerned about how she going to adjust to her mother dying. Meanwhile, Jenny's son, Andrew, has a strained relationship with his parents. He is torn between his mum and his wife and this can complicate matters.

When looking after families like Jenny's, it is important to encourage them to talk openly and honestly with each other. If Jenny and Stephen are unsure how to talk to their children or where to start, you can work with them so they can rehearse what they want to say and how they are going to say it. They may ask you to be with them when they do. Even though they have different relationships with their children, the best advice is to tell them exactly the same information and, if possible, at the same time. It also helps to spend time with their children, allowing them to ask questions and decide as a family how they move forward. Not all relationships are close, for example, Andrew may feel sad about his mother and upset about the strained relationship he has had with her of late. It is important to be aware of family members who may have a complicated bereavement and offer them information about bereavement support after the death.

Parents

A mother or father will always want to parent and care for their child, no matter what the age of the child. To lose a child as an adult is a particularly hard loss, but the needs of an elderly parent are often forgotten when their adult child is dying. They may feel helpless and a burden themselves at such a difficult time for the family. Many feel guilt that it isn't them who is dying rather than their child.

Jenny's mum, Freda

Freda doesn't want to be a burden to her daughter and her family so she tells them she's fine, no need to visit her, she is well looked after. In her haste to care for her daughter and not be a burden, she feels isolated and alone and feels others may think it unfair that she is still alive while her child is dying. But including her in the family allows her to feel involved and able to say goodbye to her child.

Elderly bereaved parents can experience great loss that goes unnoticed. So what could you do to support Freda? First, she will not be protected by withholding information about Jenny, so you could talk to Jenny and Stephen about how they can discuss things with Freda and who would be the best person to support her. Involve the care home staff to ensure she has someone to talk to. They may be able to arrange to take Freda to visit Jenny. The care home staff should also consider the bereavement phase as losing an adult child can result in a complex and long-term phase of bereavement.

Many family members, whether a partner, adult child or parent, willingly take on the role of carer. They want to do all that they can for the person that they love and often see themselves as the best person to do this. They do, however, need to be encouraged to take time to just 'be' with the person that is dying; to remember that they are a husband or a daughter first and a carer second. Some of the people who choose to die at home may elect to have a short **respite** stay in a hospice. This may be so that family carers can have a rest, but also so that, for the period of the respite care, they can go back to being the husband or wife or daughter.

Young children

Children can feel confused by the many changes that occur when someone in their family is dying. This could be due to more professionals being around or extra equipment at home. Children like routine, so when Jenny can no longer pick her grandchildren up from school, or undertake tasks she used to do, it can be a distressing experience. Children may not be able to verbalise their distress or sadness. Instead they may play it out in different behaviour; becoming withdrawn, being naughty or challenging decisions.

It is crucial to reassure the child or young person that though things are changing, all will be done to try and minimise the disruption to their world. Continuing a normal routine and the use of previous boundaries and areas of behavioural management will help children feel secure in a changing environment. Children may misbehave at these times but it is important to avoid telling children to behave as adults. Avoid common sayings such as 'You are the man of the house now' or 'Be good for Daddy' as they need to be able to express how they are even though this may be through challenging behaviour. Most importantly, they need the reassurance that they are loved and cared for and this will not change.

Adults will naturally want to do everything they can to protect children from finding out about upsetting or sad news and think that withholding information is protecting them. But children do need to be told. Children as young as a few months old will be aware that things are different and, while parents may feel they are protecting them from what is happening, it is likely that the child has already realised that there is something wrong. Children are alert to anything different, they may witness subtle changes in behaviour, whispered conversations or a shift in atmosphere, and so often they know something is wrong. Children can fear the death of their parent as they witness changes in how they look or behave, even if death is not imminent or they have not been told the parent will die. This may mean their imagination runs away with them when the reality may be easier to cope with.

Children: different needs at different ages

The people that we care for will often have children in their lives – these may be their own children, grandchildren, even great-grandchildren. We know that children of different ages will understand and behave in different ways and this is a guide to what children will understand:

- *Babies and toddlers* will notice that a parent or carer is not around as much, is sleeping or too tired to play. They may also be spending time with alternative caregivers as the parent or carer is too unwell to care for the child, even when they are at home. The shift in familiar people or routine can be disruptive to babies.

- *Primary school-aged children* will notice physical changes such as a person losing their hair, being fatigued or suffering reduced mobility. They will also notice emotional changes such as adults being tearful, talking in hushed voices or changes in their routine.
- For *teenagers*, all of the above will happen, but they will also be in a position where they may know what words such as 'hospice' or 'cancer' means. If they do not know, they will use the internet to look it up. Searching on the internet can be informative, but it can also provide a million different explanations for a situation which can be very scary for a teenager to read if they do not know the reality of what is happening for their family member.

We know that children adjust and cope better after the death of a family member if they are prepared for it. Depending on their age, children may ask difficult questions or they may withdraw. In order for all of the family to adjust and cope, honest but gentle communication, in ways children will understand (depending on their age), is needed. One of Jenny's grandsons lives 200 miles away and doesn't have the same relationship with his grandmother as the other two, but he too needs to understand what is happening and have the opportunity to see his grandmother if he wishes. If he is not prepared, he may experience problems after his grandmother dies; lost opportunities, or confusion about why he doesn't know her well. These things could affect his grief.

The parents should be involved in telling the children. It may be that they need to be supported in how to talk to their children or the parents prefer to be with you when you talk to them, but the parents need to be prepared and rehearse what they are going to say in a quiet place and protected time.

The following provides some practical tips on how to communicate with children:

- *The language used.* Always use the correct words for what is wrong with the person, for example, they have cancer, they have motor neurone disease. Many charities specific to particular illnesses produce leaflets which help explain the illness to children. Some of these are listed at the end of the chapter. Despite the temptation to avoid them, it's important you use the words 'die' and 'death' rather than 'pass on', 'go to sleep' or other terms that make death sound nicer.

- *Timing.* Avoid telling a child everything in one sitting. Children like to go back and reflect on what they have been told and then come back to ask questions when they are ready. Be prepared for questions and give honest answers in language the child will understand and check their understanding each time.
- *Honesty.* Don't give false hope. Untruths will be revealed as the dying person deteriorates and can affect trust between the children and the adults. If a person has been told that they have a short prognosis, it is better for a child to be aware that their time with the person may be limited so that they have the oppor- tunity to say goodbye and to talk to them or do activities with them to make memories. Some of these are listed in the Appendix.

It is important to reassure the children about what will happen after the person has died. This includes things such as where they will live, who will look after them, whether they will be able to continue going to the same school and if they will still be able to see friends. These are all really important things for children, and may be things that they are really worried about but do not want to ask. Children need to be reassured that, whatever happens, there will always be people to love them and look after them.

Remember it is OK to say 'I don't know.' Children may ask questions to which there is no answer. In situations such as this, it is fine to say you don't know.

Working with others

You may wish to work with the parents or grandparents to prepare answers for the child's questions and ensure everyone in the family is saying the same thing. People often want professionals to tell the children what is wrong as they do not feel able to do it themselves. Find out why they don't want to give this information – is it that they don't know what to say?, is it that they are frightened as to how the child will react? or is it simply that they do not want to upset the child? All of these reservations can be explored; it is, however, usually better for a parent or carer to tell a child what is happening themselves. They know the individual needs of the child best. Often there will be a shared history – 'Do you remember when Grandma was in hospital?' It also allows the child to feel confident to go back and ask more questions when they feel ready. For the person telling the child, it is important that they are supported in telling the children, either by family or friends or professionals such as nurses, social workers or therapists.

What happens if children are not told what is happening?

Some families decide not to tell children what is happening, this is often because they want to protect the child and not cause them distress. The decision that a family makes concerning this should be respected, however, not telling a child what is happening can have consequences.

Children, even very young children, will make up their own version of what is happening if they are not told. This can often be even worse than the reality, however bad that may be. Older children may feel cheated of the opportunity to say goodbye properly to the person who is unwell, and may feel resentful to the parent who is left for keeping information from them. This can lead to difficult relationships moving forward. Children may blame themselves for the person being unwell. They may feel that the person is unwell because they have not been doing well at school or because they have been very naughty. Children may be fearful that they can catch the illness and may die themselves, or that all of the people around them will die. Children may feel that they are not considered important enough to be told what is happening.

It is important that everyone involved with the children is aware of the situation. This may include talking to the child's nursery, school or seeking specialist advice from nurses, social workers or a therapist.

It can be challenging to help families to communicate with each other. There are many resources to help you talk to families and families to talk to their children listed in the Appendix at the end of this book. The importance of effective communication was previously discussed in **Chapter 4**. It may be useful to look at this to help you to help families to communicate with each other.

Jenny and her grandchildren

Jenny and Stephen had spoken over the last year of her life about preparing their family and sought support in doing so with the specialist palliative care nurse.

They talked over how to communicate with Sarah and Andrew and ways to prepare the grandchildren and what activities may be useful in helping the grandchildren cope. Jenny had prepared memory boxes for all three of her grandchildren to have when she died but struggled with telling them she was dying. Sarah and Stephen also struggled to tell them. But the children knew something was wrong, Grandma slept a lot, stopped picking them up from school. They overheard whispered telephone conversations and saw worried glances between adults.

What could you do to support Sarah and Andrew? From what you have read in this chapter, think about how you would help them talk to their children about their grandmother and prepare them for her death.

Ultimately, each situation and each child is different and it is important to adapt language and approach accordingly. It can feel that you are being overly honest; the reality is children need an opportunity to understand and manage information in order to process that information.

In this chapter we have talked about the needs of individuals within a family and how you can support them. There may be others who have an important role with the dying person, such as friends or work colleagues. The relationship between friends and work colleagues can be very close. They may have known the person who is dying for many years and, as someone caring for the dying person, you may come into contact with their friends and/or work colleagues. The same principles that we have discussed above apply to them in communicating and supporting those who are significant to the dying person.

All too often, healthcare workers find this area of their practice so challenging that they do nothing. It can be difficult but by introducing the question about how families would like to communicate and offering your support and the information they need, you can help a family both cope with the process of someone dying within the family and help them adjust and cope better after the person has died. Your role in this could be pivotal in enabling families to work together, talk to each other and support each other. This will influence how the person who is dying and the family approach the inevitable death and how the family grieve afterwards.

A multiprofessional team approach

Remember you are a part of a wider team and there will be others who can help you support families. In particular, social workers have experience in working with families of people of all ages. Other members of the team may be useful, for example, the clinical nurse specialist or GP may be able to explain the illness and its consequences to the family in a way that can best help them to understand and plan together.

Activities to help prepare children for the death of a parent or grandparent

Memory box

A memory box is a positive way for the person who is dying to collate information and mementos of their life that can be shared with their children either before or after their death. This can include a journal which provides a story of the person's life. This may include details of the person's childhood, their adult life, details of family and friends, memories of their children growing up as well as documenting their hopes for the children's future. It is important that the parent is not too ambitious for their child. If they do not achieve what their parent wanted for them, they may feel they have let them down.

The memory box could also include personal belongings such as items of clothing or jewellery, cards or pictures that the children had made for the person and items which remind them of special times such as a pebble from a family holiday or a perfume which brings back memories of a special time. If a person has died very suddenly, an adult can support a child to make a memory box in which they can put in important things that remind them of the person who has died. A memory book or photobook is another way of doing this.

Letters, cards, videos

Many people want to leave a special message for their children to read or listen to after they have died. This could include a letter or birthday cards for special occasions. People may also choose to record a message so that children have a visual and audio memory of the person who has died. It is important when leaving messages to avoid phrases such as 'I am leaving you in charge' or 'you are now responsible' for something or someone. Using words such as these can place a level of pressure and responsibility onto a child which they may try to achieve, yet their maturity and age may not allow this. This in turn can lead to them feeling that they have failed the person who has died. As a result, letters to children should provide positive and realistic hopes for the future as well as positive reflections on the past. If someone is very unwell and is only able to write for short periods of time, note cards with heading such as 'My hope is …', 'My favourite memory of you is …' can help them to think about what they want to say. This allows for short but focused thoughts which the person can leave for family members.

Drawing

For some children, the idea of sitting down and telling someone how they are feeling is very daunting as they may not understand themselves how they are feeling or may not know the words to describe these feelings. Allowing children to draw a picture of their situation is a simple way to engage a child. Once a picture has been drawn, an adult can ask the child to tell them what the picture represents. This often enables the child to describe their feelings in a safe way as they feel they are talking about the picture and not themselves. When a person is dying, a child may want to draw a card or picture which they can give to the person. If the child wishes, this picture can be put in the coffin with the person following the death so that something of the child remains with the deceased.

Worry dolls

These can be used with children both before and after the parent's or grandparent's death. Traditionally, worry dolls come from an Indian legend which suggested that children should share their worries with the doll before they go to sleep. The doll is then the keeper of the worry and is placed under the pillow to stop the child worrying and to enable them to have a peaceful sleep. Dolls are often sold in a small fabric bag with six dolls. This allows for up to six worries to be shared. They can be bought online. Children may also want to make their own dolls using wooden pegs or pipe cleaners.

Memory or feelings jars

The aim of the activity is to fill a jam jar with different coloured salt to represent memories of the person who has died. It can also be made to represent feelings about the person who is dying or has died. The equipment needed is very limited and includes: a clean empty jam jar with a lid, coloured chalks, and sheets of paper, a label for the jar, cotton wool and salt.

- Carefully fill the jar with salt and place to one side.
- On the label ask the child to write down any four memories of the person who died/how they are feeling at that time (this can be a good conversation tool).
- Draw a dot of colour next to each memory (for example, blue for their favourite song).
- Spread out four sheets of paper and split the salt from the jar between them.
- Colour each pile of salt one of the colours of the dots by rubbing a piece of coloured chalk into it.
- Pour each pile of salt into the jar one at a time to create memories/ feelings. Fill up any remaining space with cotton wool to stop moisture getting in the jar.
- Attach a tag to the jar and decorate as you wish.

Feelings picture

There are a large number of activity sheets available which show the various emotions that we feel. If a child is finding it hard to talk about their feelings, showing pictures of various faces with different emotions can be a good starting point to help them to explore how they are feeling.

 Where to find more information

All these activities and further advice can be found online. There are suggested websites together with some books that may help children of different ages in the resources section in the Appendix at the end of this book.

This chapter has explored the impact a life-threatening illness can have on a family. Each family is unique and as carers we are invited in for a short time. We must not assume or try to change family dynamics but be respectful of and sensitive to them.

Helping families: things to remember

- We all have different roles and relationships and these can change as someone close to us approaches death.
- The different roles should be acknowledged and respected.
- Honest discussion within a family should be encouraged.
- There are many tools, books and professionals that can help people explore the imminent loss of someone they care about.

 Individuals all have attitudes, values and beliefs. Some of these will be shared, but in some families opposing attitudes and beliefs may be present. **Chapter 8** will consider how beliefs can influence a person's dying.

How do people's beliefs, values and attitudes influence their dying?

*Roz Claydon, Helen Healey,
Irene Webster and Clair Sadler*

This chapter will

- explore some of our attitudes and beliefs and how these can shape views about death and dying;
- consider different ways in which these attitudes and beliefs can be expressed.

Can you imagine what would be a good death for you? How old would you be? Think about the situation. Who would you choose to have with you? What are they doing? Where are you? Have you had time to think about what you want?

An exercise like this can feel scary but it is important that we think about these things as they shape who we are and help us think how we can care for others at this time. In **Chapter 2** we considered advance care planning, providing the opportunity for someone to think about what they want when they die. Giving the person who is dying, space and time to explore their thoughts and feelings about dying can be hard but equally rewarding.

Beliefs, values and attitudes: what are they and why is it important to know?

As people, we all have beliefs, values and attitudes about the things that are important to us. These can be shaped by our upbringing, our experiences, the culture in which we live, and where we live. Beliefs, values and attitudes shape a person and impact greatly on the way that a person lives their life and often the way in which they die. This chapter will explore why it is important to acknowledge and respect what a person believes, ways to explore this and practical issues to consider.

Beliefs are what we think about ourselves and our place in the world. They are frequently very deep-seated and it is often hard for us to remember where they first came from. *Values* are about how we have concluded things ought to be or people ought to behave, especially in terms of qualities such as honesty, dignity, respect and kindness. *Attitudes* are how we respond to people and situations based on the beliefs and the values that we hold and that they hold.

We are in a privileged position when we are with someone as they approach the end of their life. As a carer, we should consider the idea that all people have an equal right to care, that we value dignity as central to all the care we deliver and hold the attitude that everyone we care for deserves respect and care at the end of their life, who-ever they are and whatever their beliefs and values. Beliefs, values and attitudes are often very deep-seated, and we can be unaware of them. They are so much part of who we are that if we want to help someone explore how they feel, it is vital that we have insight into what is important to us as individuals. This insight will influence the care that we are able to give someone at the end of their life.

How do we know what we value in life? Perhaps we only fully under-stand when it becomes certain it is coming to an end. This is often the case for the people that we are caring for. What we value, what we are attracted to and what is important to us may be magnified when we face death.

People facing death often have a new sense of clarity. The day-to-day chaos of life is swept aside. When the aeroplanes were flown into the Twin Towers in New York in the 9/11 terrorist attack, what did the people in the burning towers do first? Many phoned those who were important to them and said 'I love you.'

Spirituality and religion: are they different?

The terms 'spirituality' and 'religion' are often used interchangeably but are distinctly different. Spirituality can be defined as the way in which we know ourselves, what makes us unique, our way of making sense of our beliefs, values and attitudes. Quite simply, spirituality is being human. Religion can be a way that some people choose to express this. This expression can be purely personal but more commonly as a collective and recognised corporate belief system, or devotion to something outside ourselves, a higher being. Religion, for many people, can guide the way in which they live.

Central to the care that we offer is connecting as a human with another human. To do this, we need to be aware of who we are and what makes us tick – this includes an awareness and care of people's spirituality and religious convictions.

Spirituality in healthcare

Although we meet the person in our specific role as carer, what is sometimes needed is the ability to step outside of this role and simply be with the person. Some examples that come to mind are: a nurse taking delight and pride in her ability to do a patient's nails, hair and make-up and the importance and value this had for patients, a carer singing for a patient, laughing together, or a moment of tears and shared sadness.

These words from a nurse working in a hospice sum this up:

> Reflecting on what patients at the end of life want from us as carers, I have thought of the patients I care for. I have noticed how patients who are dying gradually lose interest in the world and seem to withdraw. Patients near the end of life also seem to be less concerned about their body and what is happening to it. At the end of life, relationships, love, and contact with others undergo changes. It is almost that, as the patient weakens, the things of most value are transformed into symbols. So a picture of loved ones, a blanket from home, flowers from the garden have a meaning far beyond what we can see. It is the same with our care. Small acts of kindness, comforting, and ensuring the patient is as comfortable and as peaceful as possible also communicate, symbolically, that they are loved and cared for.

It is recognised in health and social care that spirituality is a topic that is difficult to discuss and is up there with sexuality as a topic that a lot of us would choose to avoid talking about. This reluctance could be for a number of different reasons: lack of confidence to raise the topic, feeling that it is a very private topic best avoided or not that relevant. Carers sometimes argue that it is the physical needs of the person that are important, not what they believe in. Another recurring barrier is that someone will say, 'I have known the person for some time and as they approach the end of their life it is too late, or it would be inappropriate to raise such issues at this stage because it would upset them.' The counter-argument to this is that it is never too late. While there is a risk that we may cause distress, handled sensitively, significant conversations can be had. Experience would suggest that these discussions can take place when we first meet someone. See **Chapter 4** on how to carry out these conversations.

The focus of this book is that **end of life care** is everybody's business – sometimes we can feel that there is someone else that is better equipped to have these conversations, or we may hear someone say: 'It is not my job.' But a person's belief system is so central to who they are that it is the business of everyone who looks after them. It may be that the person wants very practical help – help to arrange the visit of a friend or a faith leader. It may be that they are frightened and want someone to sit with them or just hold their hand. We will only know if we are prepared to listen to them.

Respecting someone as an individual

Spiritual needs, especially at the end of life, should be considered equally alongside physical needs. People nearing the end of life may be less concerned about their body and what is happening to it.

In **Chapter 5** we discussed ways of assessing the needs of a person and the impact that pain or other symptoms can have on a person's life (and potential death). A person can also experience pain in many ways, one of which is spiritual pain. As with more physical aspects of pain, there are formal models and tools to assess people's spiritual needs. However, there are also some very practical, intuitive ways in which this can be done. Many of these will be done when we first meet a person but they will most probably evolve over time as we get to know the person better.

It can be useful to know who is around the person, who is doing what and what their significance is to them. This can be by working out a very simple family tree.

Maria's family tree

Maria is 78 years old and married to Aldo. She had eight brothers and sisters, all older than her. She has one brother who still who lives in Italy, they have lost contact over recent years. Maria and Aldo have three children – Angelo, Lily and Nancy – they are all married and have three children each. Angelo and his family now live in the USA and visit annually, and the regular phone conversations have reduced as Maria is increasingly hard of hearing. Lily and Nancy manage the family restaurant, live locally and visit daily. Maria has a goddaughter, Tessa, the daughter of her childhood friend. Since Tessa's mother died when Tessa was 21, they have become very close and Tessa looks on Maria as a second mother.

This very simple insight into Maria and her family gives us many pointers that may affect Maria and what she wants as she approaches the end of her life. Would contact with her brother help her – are there things she wants to say to him? Does she want more contact with Angelo and his family – would Skype be an option to facilitate this? Would we have known about how important Tessa was to Maria if we had just asked about her children? This information can be gained from direct questioning with Maria but equally it may be through incidental conversations, by sitting and looking through photos that she may have, talking with Maria and her husband and family developing a picture of who Maria is and what is important to her.

Hobbies and activities

Many of the people that we care for have declining health and mobility and may not be able to actively engage in activities. The person may still be very interested, for example, the man who can no longer get to the football match but wants to listen to the football results each Saturday teatime, as he always has, the retired tree surgeon who has his bed moved so that he can see the grand oak tree in the garden or the woman who loves to have her jazz CD playing and a gin and tonic at 5 p.m. each day. These are simple examples of how we can help the person approaching the end of their life maintain their identity and simple ways by which we can respect who they are.

Organisations

There are also organisations that help people who are approaching the end of their life to live out what is important to them.

Animal lovers may benefit from a visit from a volunteer from Pets as therapy, or similar charities. Volunteers take their pets, usually dogs, into care homes, hospitals, hospices, day centres, schools, etc. The power of such visits can be seen in the work of Bill, the black Labrador.

Albert and Bill, the black Labrador

Bill, the black Labrador visited Albert on a regular basis over a period of 12 months in the care home where he lived. Albert had had dogs all his life since childhood and he loved them. He had dementia but, when lucid, would remember and talk about Bill's visits and looked forward to the next one. When Albert was unwell and bed-bound, Bill would sit by his bed wagging his tail and Albert would look at him and smile.

Bill also visited Alice in the care home. As a result of her dementia, she had lost the ability to talk but her carers knew she had always loved animals. When Bill visited, she would become very excited and unclench her fists and loved Bill to drool over her hands. While Alice was approaching the end of her life, this simple act appeared to take her back to a former time.

Visits can take different forms. You may wish to access the moving clip of 'Gladys', a lady with advanced dementia, see the Appendix.

Religion

An individual's religion can be little more than a label, a statement that they put on official documents. In the 2011 census, 59.3 per cent of the British population stated that they were Christian. The percentage of the British public with an active Christian faith, however, is much lower. Religion, however, can be an extremely important part of many people's lives and is the way that they express their spirituality and who they are. Religious expression is rarely a totally solitary act. Religion is about believing in a higher being at an individual level but also often about belonging to a religious group. A Christian may be an active member of a specific parish, whereas celebrating Shabbat with family can be an important part of the life of a Jew, and for a Muslim, visiting their local mosque and the call to prayer are a significant part of who they are and how they live. It can be our role to help an individual express this in whatever way is appropriate and possible. Some people may have a dormant faith and request contact with a faith leader as they approach the end of their life – this request is usually possible to accommodate.

As someone approaches the end of their life, they may be comforted (or daunted) by their beliefs. It is important to acknowledge that not everyone has a religion, but someone with no religious faith can still have spiritual needs.

Skills of addressing spiritual needs

As was discussed earlier, one of the main ways we can identify an individual's 'spiritual need' is through our communication with them.

 In **Chapter 4** we considered communication in depth and the different approaches we may use. Simple questions that could be asked in this context could be:

- Would you like to talk to someone about how you are feeling?
- Who do you think might be able to help?
- What or who do you feel helps you when you have had a difficult time in your life?

Such questions can open up a conversation and help the person feel that they have permission to talk about the things that are important to them.

Many people at the end of their life want to focus on their relationships and may need to be encouraged to say the following to those significant to them:

- I love you.
- Thank you.
- I am sorry.

Such statements are deeply personal, very important and can be difficult for people to express. Part of our job can be to provide 'space' for these conversations to happen. It may be that certain people should not be present – encouraging a wife to leave the room so that a father can talk to his son, for example. This may not be easy but it is very important.

Sometimes it is more appropriate to express these things in an alternative way – a letter that they write or dictate, or a video recording of the person saying what they want to say. All of which we can help with, if required.

Spiritual pain

We covered physical pain in **Chapter 5**. Spiritual pain can be harder to detect, assess and treat than its physical counterpart. Physical pain can be made worse if there is a spiritual dimension that is not managed and, vice versa, unrelieved physical pain may in itself lead to spiritual and emotional pain.

Pain can be compared to an iceberg. The tip that is visible above the surface of the water is the physical pain, that is what the world sees. However, under the surface, it can be much more. This can be the spiritual and emotional element of suffering. It is not always visible and can take time and effort to explore. It could be related to many things – vulnerability, fear of death – what happens at death and what will happen after death, or anxiety, conflict, guilt, unfinished business, feeling of abandonment by family or a higher being.

How can we detect spiritual pain and what can be done to help?

Spiritual pain can be difficult to 'diagnose'. As with physical symptoms, there may be signs that the individual is experiencing spiritual pain such as:

- restlessness and agitation
- withdrawal
- anger
- sleeplessness
- not wanting to be a 'burden'.

Identifying the problem is the first stage to findng to a solution. Often spiritual pain is related to physical issues that, once resolved, can improve. Sometimes the reason for the pain is that the person is in turmoil inside and we could have a role in helping them deal with their fears or bad feelings or whatever is troubling them. They may have unfinished business that we can help them sort out. Would it help if the person met a solicitor to change their will? Is there someone that they need to see or contact? Some spiritual pain is related to a religious component, the need for forgiveness from a higher being and this may be the only way of putting things right. For some faiths, the provision of the last rites or a blessing is vital when death is imminent.

Maria's faith

Maria takes great comfort from her Catholic faith. Her parish priest visits regularly and administers Holy Communion on a weekly basis and listens to her confession as she wishes. She is accepting of her imminent death and feels that her faith has helped with this. Her greatest sadness, however, is that her son Angelo lives in America. She misses him and wonders if she will see him again before she dies. Her goddaughter found her crying and, after some coaxing, she told Tessa her fear. Tessa explained about Skype to Maria and arranged to bring her tablet round to Maria's house to set it all up. Maria was able to see and talk to Angelo which gave them both great comfort and she told him how much she loved him. The Skype conversations made Angelo realise how unwell his mother was and he flew home to spend the final two weeks of her life with her.

Living and working in a multicultural society

As previously stated much of what we believe comes from the culture in which we were brought up or live. The United Kingdom is an increasingly multicultural society so those requiring care and those offering care can be from a vast array of different countries, cultures and belief systems. This can at times lead to conflict and can be challenging.

It is beyond the remit of this book to offer precise direction on the cultural needs of different people. We would suggest, however, that if you are caring for a person who has a different culture or belief system than your own that you explore this by answering the questions listed below. These questions can be answered by the person, their families, other staff who have a similar belief systems or by contacting the relevant organisation/or place of worship if appropriate.

Think about the different cultures and religious backgrounds of the people you care for. Do you know what the different customs and ceremonies are for each as their condition deteriorates and when they die?

- Are there are any last rites or rituals that need to be performed before the person dies?
- When the person is dying, are there people who need or want to be in attendance?
- Immediately after the person has died, who should care for the body? It is important to consider who should wash or dress them. Does it have to be a family member, religious leader or can it be the person who has cared for them?
- Is there a time period in which the body needs to be moved to the funeral directors/burial site/place of worship?
- If someone dies on a religious day, such as a Jewish person on the Sabbath, what happens?

What we believe and how it can impact on the people we care for

We all have beliefs, values and attitudes, whether we are the carer or the person being cared for. For some people, these beliefs can be the reason why they chose to work in a caring job. What a person believes will obviously shape the care that they deliver. It is vital that as carers, whether qualified or not, all our actions are guided by the person that we are caring for. This is as true for spiritual care as any other aspect. A person may ask us what we believe – this is very different from imposing our values on the person. While it may be tempting to share what is important to us, we must always handle such conversations with sensitivity and respect for the other person. Any discussion should be with the person's consent and it may be that there are local policies or codes of practice that we work within. At times, we may need to put aside our own beliefs. The carer may find this hard and may need support themselves at this time.

Helping a person to deal with their feelings can be difficult, particularly as they near the end of their life. It can be draining, daunting or make us sad and this can be the reason why sometimes we choose not to discuss some of these very important issues. We should be aware of this and think of strategies that may help us to deal with this aspect of the care that we offer. **Chapter 11** offers some practical guidance for help for carers.

Showing respect and treating with dignity

This chapter has identified how a person's beliefs, values and attitudes influence their dying. As carers it is vital that we acknowledge the things that make them 'who they are'. We do this through our respect for them as an individual and respecting their spirituality. The list that follows gives some of the ways in which we show someone that we respect them. Some things on the list may seem very natural, others less so. It is worth checking and asking yourself from time to time, 'Do I do these things and, if not, why don't I?' Ask yourself, 'Do I avoid these difficult conversations and why?' Is it that you do not feel comfortable or are you worried about how the conversation may go? What can you do to 'stay with' the person who is dying while they talk to you?

● *Space.* We do not always look after people in an 'ideal environment', whether in an institution or their own home. There can be lots of noise and activity and we need to be aware of the impact this can have on someone's ability to express what is important to them.

● *Privacy.* In the same way, privacy, despite some of the challenges, should be respected. Do we knock before we enter their room? Are they embarrassed during personal care? Are there ways that they can have time on their own or with people significant to them without being disturbed?

● *Individuality.* At the heart of helping someone is the acknowledgement that they are an individual with individual needs. We need to help them express this and their wishes should be respected. In order that we can best do this, we need to know what is important to the person.

● *Ritual and tradition.* Spirituality and religion are not the same thing. Many people, however, express themselves though their faith. This may be the way that they dress, for example, Sheikh men may wear turbans or Muslim women may wear hijabs or burkas. Alternatively, it may be the way that they worship, for example, meditation is central to the Buddhist faith, this could take place in a temple or may be at a shrine set up in the person's home. Matters concerning food are significant in many faiths, whether this be fasting or celebratory meals such as at Diwali or the Jewish Sabbath. For others, religion is not a central part of their lives but there are still important rituals significant to them, for example, it may be their role within a family and this can be challenged at a time of serious illness. We need to be sensitive and responsive to this.

- *Accessing support.* The majority of the care that we offer is as part of a wider team. This will involve healthcare and social care and voluntary services. It is important to know what is available in the local area and how services can be accessed so that we can be as responsive as possible to the people that we are caring for.

Finally, it is important to remember: it's never too late to help someone express who they really are and what is important to them.

> Somebody should tell us, right at the start of our lives, that we are dying. Then we might live life to the limit, every minute of every day. Do it! I say. Whatever you want to do, do it now! There are only so many tomorrows.
>
> (Pope Paul VI, Italian Pope, 1897–1978)

People's beliefs, values and attitudes and why they are important: things to remember

- A person's beliefs, values and attitudes are at the heart of who they are and can take on an increased significance as they approach the end of their life.
- Expression of spirituality is important and many simple things can be done to help someone express this – should they wish to.
- Has the person that you care for had the opportunity to say 'thank you', 'I am sorry' and 'I love you' to the people who are important to them?

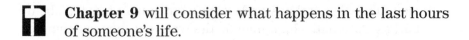 **Chapter 9** will consider what happens in the last hours of someone's life.

How to care for someone in the last hours of their life

Karen Cook, Sue Dunlop and Clair Sadler

This chapter will explore:

- signs that may suggest that someone is approaching the last hours of their life;
- choices that a person may make regarding the last hours of their life

> The last part of life may have an importance out of all proportion to its length.
>
> (Dame Cicely Saunders)

This quote from the founder of the modern hospice movement highlights how important it is to 'get it right' when someone is imminently dying, regardless of their place of death. In **Chapter 5** and **Chapter 6** we looked at some of the symptoms that may be experienced by a person as they approach their death. This chapter will consider their needs and care as they enter the final hours of their life. These 'hours' could extend into a few days and are usually referred to as the terminal phase.

Most people may not have witnessed someone's death. It can be a frightening prospect particularly if they do not know what to expect. These last days and hours can be stressful and upsetting for the dying person, and those caring for them – whether the giving of care is part of their job or it is a friend or family member that is dying. Understanding what will happen and what may help can be useful. This chapter will consider some of the common indicators that death may be close; it will describe these signs and symptoms focusing on how you may be able to help support the person and those closest to them. Symptom management, comfort measures and communication are crucial at any point in the person's illness but may be heightened at this stage of their lives. It is important because those close to the person will have to continue after the death with these memories. As Saunders (1989) said: 'How people die remains in the memory of those who live on.'

 Different illnesses and conditions follow different patterns and in **Chapter 1** we looked at some of these patterns. It can be difficult to predict exactly when someone is going to die but there are some frequently seen signs that may lead us to believe that the person is entering the last hours of their life. A knowledge of the person is vital at any stage in their illness. You may have known them for some time or only briefly. Whichever is the case, finding out about them and the ongoing assessment of their needs and what they want is important.

Think about what you know about the people you are caring for. What and who is important to them? What would they want and expect at this stage in their lives?

Before we can provide the appropriate care at this stage of someone's life, the 'team' looking after the person should agree that they are entering the terminal phase. The team may consist of many different people who have been involved in the person's care; but also possibly the person themselves. It is not uncommon for a person to 'diagnose' themselves as dying, stating that they think this is the case so it is important that this should be acknowledged.

Albert's last hours of his life

Albert's condition is deteriorating. He is increasingly unresponsive. He no longer opens his eyes or makes a noise. He is producing very small amounts of urine but he lost control of his bladder a week ago; he is lying on pads and they need regular changing. He is generally calm but gets agitated and grimaces if he is positioned on his right side. He settles quickly though if care is taken over the position he is placed in. His hands are cold to the touch and have a blue tint to them and his mouth tends to stay open. Albert's breathing has been noisy and his chest has sounded bubbly for a couple of days but now his breathing seems shallow and there are longer gaps between breaths. His closest relative, his niece Jackie, has been visiting regularly; she has said that she wants to be with him when he dies if possible, so she is called, despite it being midnight.

Albert died very peacefully two hours after Jackie arrived. She stayed with him for a short time to say her goodbye.

Albert's experience is not uncommon – another person may experience some, all or none of these things but knowledge of them may help you to know what to look out for so that you can identify that this is the terminal phase and therefore tailor the care to the needs of the individual. If we recognise that the person is dying imminently, then certain decisions may need to be discussed. Friends and family members will need time and support from you, with explanations about what is happening to their relative and why. What appears obvious to those responsible for care may be new and scary to someone who has never seen someone dying before; keep them informed of what is happening to prepare them for the death. This chapter will look in more detail at some of the signs of death being close and will detail practical ways that we can offer to help. The signs that will be discussed are:

- withdrawing from the world;
- taking reduced food and fluids;
- changes in the person's breathing;
- visions, restlessness and confusion;
- managing pain and other symptoms.

The chapter will also look at some of things we need to remember when looking after someone who is unconscious, respecting a person's wishes and also how we can support those closest to the person.

Withdrawing from the world

As people begin to move into this last phase of their lives, they will usually become drowsy, sleeping for long periods of the day and night. Their episodes of sleep may increasingly be longer than their episodes of wakefulness. They can seem disconnected and drowsy even when they are awake. They may be unable to talk for long periods, only able to say single words or simple sentences. Gradually this sleepiness often becomes unconsciousness, where the person is unable to wake and cannot be roused. If their eyes open they may appear to have woken but are unresponsive, often with a staring expression. For some, this period of unconsciousness may carry on for several days.

What can we do to help?

The person may have family and friends that want to be with them so it is important to explain that this is a natural and gradual part of the dying process. That the person will become more sleepy and that it will reach a point when they do not awaken again.

As some people approach end of their life, they may state that they want no or very few visitors, and this can be difficult for some people to hear and will need to be handled with sensitivity.

Reduced food and fluids

Appetite gradually declines over a period of time but at this stage this can often accelerate. They may take only very small sips from drinks and small spoonfuls of food.

As with their diminishing level of consciousness, their intake will gradually worsen from a disinterest in food and drinks to an inability to swallow. This is associated with their general deterioration and weakness. They may struggle to take even a sip of water and would not be able to take their medications by mouth.

What can we do to help?

It is important to respond to the person's changing needs; if they can no longer swallow, rather than attempting to give them drinks, make sure their mouth is kept clean and moist; they may like their lips moistened with a cool (or their favourite) drink. Some people, even close to the end of their life may wish and be able to take small amounts of fluids and soft foods. This should be accommodated but this is rare and therefore our biggest role can be looking after those caring for the person who is dying. Food and life are very closely related in most people's mind and we have a natural instinct to nurture. Sometimes it is necessary to gently say to relatives that at this point food or fluids will not stop their loved one from dying.

Changes in the person's breathing

As the end of life approaches, breathing can change. Initially this may be that the person is easily out of breath – just helping them to move may leave them feeling breathless. This may not be related to any particular illness but more to do with their declining condition and the impact this is having on the person's body.

When death is approaching, you may observe more changes in their breathing. This may include Cheyne-Stokes breathing – this name is given to breathing which occurs often at the very end of life. It is often cyclical in nature, consisting of long periods where there are gaps in the person's breaths; these breaths can be interspersed with deep sighing breaths; they may be followed by a series of shallow rapid breaths.

Another potentially distressing symptom that may occur close to the end of life is noisy, moist breathing sometimes referred to as the 'death rattle'. This is due to the pooling of secretions in the windpipe and chest because of the person's deteriorating condition and their inability to take deep breaths or to cough and clear the secretions.

Opening and closing the mouth can also occur in the last hours of someone's life. This is not uncommon and relatives need to be reassured that this can be part of the changes to breathing and not a sign of hunger or thirst.

What can we do to help?

The 'death rattle' does not appear to cause the person who is dying distress but can be hard for families to hear. Family members often require an explanation and reassurance. There are some simple things that can help. Repositioning can often help lessen the impact of the secretions; try lifting the head of the bed (if it is a hospital bed) or support the person to be a little more upright by using more pillows behind their shoulders and back; if the person is unconscious, it may be more helpful to lie them almost flat while gently tilting them on to their side, using pillows to support their back and alternating the side they are lying on by changing their position.

For some people, secretions may pool in the person's mouth. This is unpleasant for the family to witness and so they will need an explanation and reassurance. Often the person remains peaceful and is not distressed. Lying the person flatter in the bed, lying the person on their side and so allowing gravity to help drain the secretions out of the mouth – they can then be wiped away gently with a cloth or mouth swabs. A towel, cloth or flannel may be placed by the head to keep clothing dry and stain-free. Suctioning the secretions is rarely appropriate as this can be distressing for the dying person, will not prevent the secretions developing and may actually lead to increased production. Occasionally suction of the oral cavity may be appropriate if, for example, a family member wants to kiss the person or the person appears distressed by the secretions. Sometimes if the person's chest sounds bubbly, medications, e.g. glycopyrronium, or hyoscine hydrobromide, can be used to try to reduce the build-up of secretions. These would need to be prescribed and given either by injection or via a **syringe pump** over 24 hours alongside other necessary drugs, giving a constant small dose. (The use of syringe pumps is explained in **Chapter 5**.) These medicines do not always work and are often more helpful if given as soon as secretions are noticed. They can prevent further build-up but not take away what is already there.

Visions, restlessness and confusion

It is not uncommon for the dying person to say they can see friends and relatives who have already died and they may even appear to be talking to them. This often brings comfort to the person who is dying and equally to their family, but can feel unusual or uncomfortable for those caring for them.

In the same way that visions can appear to be comforting, some people may hallucinate and this may lead to distress. The person may appear a little confused and not know where they are or think that they are somewhere else.

Confusion, restlessness and agitation can occur and can be very distressing. In the last hours of life the person may start fidgeting and plucking at their bed sheets or even trying to get out of bed. The unsettled agitation seen when a person is close to death is often referred to as 'terminal restlessness'.

What can we do to help?

There may be a simple reason why the person is restless. The reasons could include: pain, anxiety, a feeling that they have unfinished business, a full bladder, a full rectum, metabolic changes related to their deterioration or related to their medications. For some of these reasons, there may not be a solution – changes may be occurring because of the dying process itself and may not be reversible. It is, though, worth checking the more simple causes – when did they last pass urine? Do they need 'permission' to pass urine into a pad? Would they benefit from a catheter to drain their urine? Who could you ask to assess this? If they haven't had their bowels open for a while, would it be appropriate to give laxatives? Or would it be better to manage the discomfort that they are experiencing by using painkillers? Are they lying in an uncomfortable position?

Look for obvious causes first. Talk to family members to see if there is anything they are aware of that may cause the person to be restless. If they have been looking after the dying person for a while, they may be able to understand what different behaviour means.

Managing pain and other symptoms

The process of dying is often the aspect that people are most scared of, rather than death itself. They may be scared of experiencing pain and other symptoms. They may have heard from others or seen in films that this is often the case – it isn't. In most cases it is possible to manage pain and other symptoms at this stage. Assessing these can be difficult when someone is in the final short days or hours of life, when they are unable to tell you verbally about their experience.

Even if the person cannot tell you in words what their pain is like, if you have knowledge of the person, you may be able to pick up on their cues. They may be frowning, groaning and restless. They may not be able to tell you but they may be able to squeeze your hand in response to simple questions. Your goal is to help the person die pain-free. Some people may refuse pain medication because they believe that the drugs will make them increasingly sleepy and hasten their death. It is important that you explain the reasons for the different medications you are using in the final days and hours and that these will neither prolong nor hasten death. Pain medication given by whatever route is calculated carefully, starting with a dose which is equivalent to the dose they would receive if still able to take by mouth. This information can be comforting to the person and their family, particularly if they have concerns about medications speeding up a person's death.

> Think about caring for someone who is experiencing pain. Even if they were able to tell you about their pain, what signs do you think might indicate that the person has uncontrolled pain or other symptoms? What expressions did they have on their face and when?

What can we do to help?

Again, as with the previous signs and symptoms, the person's family and friends may be more aware of the person's usual pain and so may notice any discrete changes. Encourage the family to let you know if they are concerned. Reassure the relatives that you are always assessing for pain and discomfort whenever you are involved with care giving, so that you can act quickly if additional medication is needed, monitoring how helpful this is and getting further advice if necessary. If the person can no longer take medicines by mouth, think about alerting their doctor or nurse so that an alternative route can be used. What other symptoms have they had in the past – have they experienced anxiety, nausea, breathlessness? Do they need replacement of oral medications given subcutaneously for these reasons? Look at **Chapter 5.**

Think about what seems to worsen or aggravate their symptoms. Some people who are dying may become stiff – this may be due to immobility while lying in one position in the bed; as with other symptoms, pain may be relieved by re-positioning. If stiffness continues and prevents comfort, painkillers and anti-anxiety medications can be given to relax the person and keep them comfortable.

Caring for someone who is unconscious

As previously stated, in the last hours of someone's life the person can become increasingly drowsy and ultimately unconscious. It is vital that we continue to care for all their needs. In the last hours of life, blood can move from the person's extremities to the vital organs. Hands and feet may feel cold and become bluer in colour, while for some the abdomen and chest can remain warm and even appear hot and sweaty. As death approaches, skin may appear mottled, the person's face may become more sunken, with their mouth falling open. Fluid may start to pool in the limbs. As blood leaves the extremities and the body begins to shut down, the pulse in the wrist weakens. The person's face may also appear yellowish or waxy – these signs, along with the changes in breathing, are often signs of imminent death.

What can we do to help?

The most important thing is to keep the person as comfortable as possible – if they are very hot, use cool clothing, remove or loosen sheets and blankets, a fan or an open window may help. Regular gentle wiping of the face with a tepid flannel is a simple act that can help maintain the person's comfort, the family may feel able to help with this. If the person has a high temperature, then medication such as paracetamol could be given. This would usually be administered via a suppository into the back passage. A decision needs to be made as to whether the administration of the medication is more or less distressing than the fever. At this stage any medication is purely a comfort measure. If the person feels cold, apply another blanket, close any windows unless specifically asked not to. Some people may have wounds that require attention. At this stage in the person's life, only change the dressing if it is wet, leaking, or to prevent an offensive odour (malodorous). Healing is no longer a goal but maintenance of comfort and dignity is. The person may require regular repositioning. This is an area where knowledge of the person, their illness and their skin integrity can make a real difference. People have to be protected from painful and unnecessary bedsores but should not be made more uncomfortable by changing their position too often if not necessary. Using pressure-relieving mattresses may reduce the amount of times a person needs to be repositioned. Tilting the person at 30 degrees using pillows is often more comfortable than turning someone right onto their side. Gauge the person's face for comfort, frowns usually mean they are uncomfortable. Some people can have very sensitive skin and may react even to the most gentle of touches; they may call out, arch their back or flinch away when touched. Be gentle even with small tasks or contacts and explain to them and their family what you are about to do. If sensitive care and reassurance are not sufficient, then it may be necessary to ask for a medical review if there are medications that may reduce the person's sensation of sensitivity.

Respecting a person's wishes

Throughout the previous chapters of this book we have discussed how important it is to know and respect what a person wants at the end of their life. This knowledge may be a gained informally by 'knowing' the person and those important to them. Increasingly, however, it is recorded formally though the process of advance care planning and shared with all those who are involved in providing care and supporting the person. In **Chapter 2** you can find out more about **advance care planning (ACP)**.

At this stage many of the people that we care for cannot be roused but this should not affect how we talk to them. They may not respond but we should still talk to them, explain what is happening.

Maria's last wishes

When she was told by her GP that there was little more that could be done to help her heart failure and that her life was very limited, she was not surprised. The GP sat with her and Aldo and talked about what they wanted as she approached the end of her life. Maria and Aldo had always made decisions together and this was not going to change now. Maria knew exactly how she wanted to die. Maria was clear she had already had three heart attacks and was adamant that she would not want to be resuscitated. Maria said she wanted to die at home. She loved her home, her family, her garden and her dog. Maria awoke in the early hours of the morning struggling to catch her breath; all the usual 'tricks' did not work. She was frightened and Aldo was frightened. In his panic he called an ambulance. The ambulance crew were unsure what they should do and with Maria and Aldo's agreement they took her to hospital where she died two days later.

Sometimes, with all the best planning and preparation, things happen and patients do not get their wishes. In this example, in the early hours of the morning Maria and Aldo were frightened and thought hospital was the best place to manage her breathlessness. Once there, her breathlessness was treated and she felt calmer and safe. An increased package of care was being developed to discharge Maria but her condition deteriorated and she became too unwell to return home.

What happened to Maria and Aldo who were so sure she would die at home? What could have been done (if anything) to ensure she died at home? What actions could you take to try and grant a person their choice of place of carer and death?

Sharing information to enable patient preferences

Maria's situation could have been different. She did not want to die in hospital but the ambulance crew that were called had little choice. This situation is not uncommon. It is hoped that electronic solutions that are being implemented across the UK will help to ensure that a person's wishes are met, if at all possible. There are geographical variations and different systems are being developed but electronic record keeping for people approaching the end of life is becoming increasingly common. The records can be accessed 24 hours a day by people involved in the person's care. The information recorded includes the diagnosis, whether the person has an advance care plan and what this plan includes.

If this had been in place, the ambulance crew that were called could have accessed this information and perhaps there would have been a different end result.

Supporting those closest to the person

Saying goodbye

People who are dying sometimes appear to need 'permission to die'. It can seem that people may wait until a specific event has happened such as news of the birth of a grandchild, for others it may be the arrival of a family member. It is equally not uncommon for someone to wait to die when everyone has left the bedside. Some friends and family may choose to be absent; some may wish to remain at the bedside continually. There may be a difference of opinion in families as to what is right, with some wanting to stay and others struggling to do so. Try not to judge those involved for their decisions, we're all different and we may not agree or behave in the same way. It is those who are left after the person has died who have to live with their decision and the memory of the person's last moments. If the person is not being cared for in their own home, we need to make provision for those close to the person to stay overnight if they choose to.

Think about a time when you and someone you are close to had to make a difficult decision where you struggled to agree. How did you feel about this? Now think about how the other person may have felt. Can you think of the reasons why they made the decision they made?

Jenny: who should be with her at the end?

Jenny is now unconscious. Her husband Stephen is sure that she can still hear and sits and talks and tells her everything that is going on in their makeshift bedroom. They have the radio playing in the background as they always had. The family understand that Jenny has only hours to live. Ten-year-old Mark asks his granddad if he can see Jenny, to say goodbye, whereas Mark's father Andrew would like to remember her as she was when she was well. Mark's mother is unsure if children should be involved with dying people, he is too young, but he is adamant. Stephen takes Mark in to say goodbye. Mark kisses Jenny, says goodbye and leaves. He is sure she can hear him even though she doesn't respond and is glad he did it and doesn't seem upset immediately. Jenny, Stephen and family are supported by Beth, the district nurse, and the palliative care nurse specialist. They started a syringe driver two days ago and have both worked hard to keep Jenny's symptoms under control.

Think about what you do in your workplace to support families. Can relatives or friends stay overnight? Is there a bed or chair for them to sleep or rest on? Do you ask the family if they want to be there at the moment when the person dies? If they don't want to be present, do they want to be telephoned whenever the person dies or would they rather wait until the next morning? Will they be on their own when they get this phone call? Who is there to support them afterwards, what services are available in your area to support bereaved families?

Think about how you might ask these questions and how you would ensure that your colleagues are also fully aware of any decisions made.

Dying alone?

We have followed the stories of Maria, Albert and Jenny. They all died with someone they loved with them. We have also learnt that some people die when their family or friends have temporarily left the room. For some of the people that we care for, however, this will not be the case. They may not have family or friends who visit. Their only contact may be with the people who care for them. When someone is known to be approaching the end of their life, team work can be important. Priorities change and it is important to ensure that a staff member can sit with the person. A colleague may have to take on additional duties for that short period. Some

 people do not want to be left alone when they are dying. See **Chapter 10** on what to do after a death and how to recognise death has occurred.

What happens when things do not go to plan?

This chapter has explored what we can do to help someone in the last hours of their life to die peacefully, in the way that they wished, to help them have a 'good death'. This is our goal but not always achievable and this can be difficult for us to accept sometimes. We may have done everything that we can but the death is not good. It is important that as every person is unique, we also remember that so is every death. Some people will die in pain, some will be restless and agitated, some people may die because they have an acute event, such as bleeding from a wound or internally. These things do happen and can be very distressing but there are two things to remember: first, more people die peacefully than don't. And, second, even if you have done everything you can to ensure that the person's wishes are honoured, sometimes events will be outwith your control and the end of life for that person will not go as planned. When this happens, take time to reflect on the challenges you experienced with colleagues and those others involved in the care so that everyone learns from the experience.

 In **Chapter 11** you can find out how we can look after ourselves as we provide care.

Caring for someone in the last hours of someone's life: things to remember

- The death of someone can be a new experience for family friends and sometimes carers – we need to support and guide people through this process.
- Knowledge of the signs of imminent death can help us tailor our care and ensure that relatives are informed.
- While most people have a 'good death', this is not always the case and we can only do our best.

 Once someone has died, there are certain practical issues that need to be considered. There can also be a significant personal cost to those caring for them and these will be addressed in **Chapter 10**.

What to do when someone dies and what to do afterwards

Clair Sadler

The deaths that we are discussing in this book are normally natural and expected. In the last chapter we considered what happens in the last hours of someone's life. This chapter will consder what happens next and will explore the following:

- saying goodbye;
- the legalities – what the law says about dying;
- how to register a death;
- cultural differences and death;
- how it feels when someone dies;
- bereavement and practical ways we can help.

There can be warning signs that the person is going to die shortly. These are not always evident but can be helpful to prepare the family. It may be that there are things that they want to say or it may be that they would like to sit with their loved one. If they have a strong faith, they may wish to ask someone from their place of worship to visit them.

Maria has died

Maria died in the Medical Assessment Unit of her local general hospital in the early hours of the morning. She had been unrousable since the previous day. In the last few hours before she died, there were increasingly long gaps between her breaths and her hands felt cold to the touch. Aldo was sitting with her holding her hand and chose to stay with her for some time after. He was calm but became concerned that she was becoming increasingly cold and asked that she should have an extra blanket.

What would you say to Aldo or his family if they asked for another blanket for Maria?

Once a person has died, there are natural processes that will occur. The person will feel increasingly cold to the touch. This is a natural process as is a gradual stiffening of the body. When the person is moved, they may still expel air that is residual in their lungs or upper respiratory tract. This can be alarming but again a natural process. There may also be some 'leakage' of urine, faeces or exudate from wounds. This should be dealt with promptly and with sensitivity as it can add to the distress of those with the person.

Caring for a person after they have died

Throughout this book we have discussed the importance of respecting people in our care and treating them with dignity. This is no different once the person has died – they are still deserving of our respect, as are their families. This will be demonstrated in the way that we care for the body, but also by thinking about the conversations that we have as we care for their needs after death, ensuring that their dignity is respected.

Despite the fact that the deaths that we are focusing on in this book are expected, the death of a loved one can still be very distressing and, despite preparation, can come as a shock to family and friends. Each death therefore needs to be treated with great sensitivity and respect.

Friends and family will often want to spend time with the person once they have died. If you are caring for the person try to make sure that they look peaceful and the area around the bed is as comfortable and tidy as possible before the body is visited. Think about, for example:

- Does the person look as comfortable as possible? They do not need to be laid flat, one or two pillows is fine.
- Do they need clean nightclothes, top sheet or pillow slip?

- Is their hair brushed (in their usual way)?
- Are their eyes shut? A little light pressure on the eyelids should ensure this.
- Are there things by the bedside that could be moved – newspapers, tissues, drinks, etc.? If available, you may choose to put some fresh flowers on the bedside or pillow.
- Is there a chair by the bedside for the visitor to sit?
- Are there any religious requests, for example, holding a rosary?

These are very simple measures that can be done very quickly but can give great comfort to a bereaved relative or friend. The memories of saying goodbye to a loved one can be long-lasting so it is important that we respect this time.

What happens when someone dies?

If a family wishes to sit with the body, or other family members who were not there at the time of death are visiting shortly afterwards, they should be warned that the body will become increasingly rigid, a natural process known as **rigor mortis**. Rigor mortis is when the body naturally becomes stiffened after death, triggered by chemical changes. It usually starts approximately 4 hours after death, is at its maximum at 12 hours and usually disappears after 24–36 hours. This is normal and natural. These timescales are only guides as it can vary from person to person, depending on age, body size and the temperature of the environment. When the body is at its most stiff, it can be difficult to move or bend limbs. Therefore, if nightwear is to be changed, this should be done sooner rather than later. This may also affect the timing of the funeral director moving the body to the funeral home. It can be reassuring for family members to know that this is only temporary so once at the funeral home, the body will be well cared for and washing and dressing will be possible.

Saying goodbye

Some relatives may find it difficult to leave; they may leave the room and return a number of times. They may require gentle encouragement to say goodbye. It can often be comforting to tell them that once the funeral director has taken the body to the funeral home, they can visit them there and spend more time saying goodbye. It should be noted that some funeral directors may charge for this if this is out of 'office hours'. Once at the funeral home, the funeral director (sometimes called undertakers) will ensure that any wishes are met, for example, the person who has died might wear specific clothes or maybe something significant is to be placed in the coffin, a book or a photo perhaps.

It is also worth noting that in the UK over 40,000 people have pacemakers fitted each year. If someone with a pacemaker wishes to be cremated, the pacemaker must be removed. This can be done in a hospital mortuary or at the funeral directors but the person organising the cremation will need to tell the undertaker.

Jenny's story – what happens next?

Jenny died peacefully at home on a Sunday afternoon. The syringe pump that had been set up by the district nurse helped with her pain and nausea and it felt to her family that she just 'fell to sleep'. When she died, Stephen called the district nurse, Beth, who arrived 30 minutes later. She confirmed that Jenny was dead and removed the syringe pump. She verified the death so that the funeral director could move her body to the funeral home. Beth explained that Jenny's GP would visit her at the funeral home and complete the death certificate the following day. Jenny's GP had been visiting Jenny regularly and had expected her to die over the weekend. The family decided not to visit her there, choosing to say goodbye at home. Her grandchildren asked whether Grandma would be allowed some 'things' in her coffin – it was agreed and each grandchild wrote a letter. Ben thought she should also have her paintbrush because she loved painting, Poppy sent her favourite hair ribbon and Mark thought a photo of the whole family on the beach would be a good idea. The funeral director obliged and three children were left feeling that they had been able to do something for their Grandma.

What the law says about someone dying

The district nurse verified that Jenny had died but, by law, death needs to be certified by a doctor. This may be done at the time of death or later, this may be at the place where the person died or at the undertakers. If there is a delay in a doctor being able to attend to confirm that the patient has died, then a nurse or paramedic who has undergone suitable training is able to verify that the person has died and this will be later certified by a doctor. The doctor or nurse will check that:

- the person is no longer breathing for at least a minute;
- they have no pulse for at least a minute;
- their eyes no longer react to light.

They will also note the time that the person has died or, if no one was there, the time that they were found. In the same way that the time of a birth can be significant for loved ones, the time of death can be equally significant. This will also appear on the death certificate. These checks will be repeated until the person verifying that the person has died is completely satisfied. Without the death being verified by an appropriate person, it is not possible for the body to be moved to the undertakers. Delays at this time can cause distress to family and carers and many district nursing services and care homes now have staff that have undergone the training required to officially verify the death.

The death should be certified by an appropriate doctor within 24 hours of the death and, at this point, a **'medical certificate of cause of death'** (MCDD) will be issued, confirming what caused the person to die. The certificate will state a primary cause of death but also issues that contributed to the death, for example, cancer of the lung and pneumonia. Old age alone, for example, would not be appropriate. This is a legal document so the doctor must write the exact cause and it is also the basis of national statistics. Handing the certificate to relatives needs to be done with sensitivity. Very occasionally, the family may not be aware of the diagnosis or underlying conditions that the deceased may have had.

What happens if the death was not expected?

If the person dies unexpectedly, in a public place, or if they might not have been seen by their family doctor in the previous 14 days, or if they have undergone recent surgery, or if the person has fallen, or if there are any suspicious circumstances, the coroner must be informed. The coroner is an independent professional, usually a lawyer or doctor who is appointed by the Crown to investigate any deaths where the circumstances are unclear or the causes are not due to natural causes. If the death is referred to the coroner, this may delay a funeral taking place. It is important to explain to relatives and friends of the person who has died that the coroner being informed does not necessarily mean that there will have to be a post mortem or inquest.

How to register death

Though you are unlikely to have to register the death of someone in your care, it is important that you have an understanding of the process involved so that you may offer the maximum support and help to bereaved relatives.

When someone dies in the United Kingdom, it is a legal requirement that a death must be registered within five days (longer if the coroner is involved). To register a death, a representative of the deceased must attend the local registry office. This representative (known as the informant) is in most cases a close relative but can also be a person who was present at the death or is taking responsibility for the funeral. Most offices have an appointment system so the informant should be encouraged to phone to book a time to attend – the death can only be registered by attending the registry office. The process usually takes about 30 minutes.

In order to register a death, and a death certificate to be issued, it is necessary to have the following information:

- full name of the person who has died including maiden name, if appropriate, and their most recent address;
- date and place of the person's death;
- date and place of birth;
- the person's occupation or previous occupation if retired;
- if the person is married, the date and place of birth of their husband/wife should be given together with their spouse's occupation;
- National Insurance number and National Insurance number of spouse or civil partner;
- Medical certificate of cause of death.

The person registering the death will be given three forms:

- Certified copies of the death certificate – the registrar will keep the original and provide the certified copies to the family. It is free to register a death but a fee is payable per copy and relatives should be advised that the cost per copy rises if they are required later. Relatives will often have to buy multiple copies as they will be required to close bank accounts, etc., and each organisation will require an original – photocopies are not usually acceptable.

- Certificate of registration/notification of death – this is free and sent to the Department of Works and Pensions, often in a pre-paid envelope provided by the registry office.
- Certificate for burial or cremation. This is also free and commonly referred to as the 'green form' and provides the funeral director with the authority to proceed with a cremation or burial.

Find out and note what services are available in your area. Do you have a list of local funeral directors and their contact details? Where is your local registry office? What is the address, phone number and opening hours? Would it be helpful if you had a leaflet, specific to your area, that you could give to family members? Are there any leaflets you could access from Age UK, for example? You should be wary of recommending a specific funeral director as this could be misunderstood so it is better for relatives to choose from those available.

 In the **Appendix**, you will find a resource section where you can find further information.

If you are caring for someone and their death is anticipated, it is important to be aware of any specific beliefs they may hold. Remember that different cultures will have different rituals and practices surrounding end of life care and the care of the body afterwards. These must be respected, accommodated and handled sensitively. It can sometimes feel difficult to ask questions about what people want when they die, but in order to respect wishes, we need to know what they are. It can make you feel uncomfortable and it can be difficult to know when the best time to do this is. It is, however, vitally important to do it so that wishes can be met.

Finding out that someone has died and how does it feel?

Think of someone you have looked after who has died. How did you learn that they had died? How did you feel? Who supported you?

Cultural differences and death

We live in a multicultural society and therefore we care for people with a range of beliefs and traditions. If we are to respect these, it is vital that we know what they are. This information may be gained on an initial meeting or by spending time with the person. Specific details and requests should be carefully recorded and communicated so that requests can be met. It is not possible to offer a complete list of rituals and traditions, because, even within a distinct religious faith, there may be different interpretations. Listed below are some key questions that you should ask when caring for someone who has a faith (religious examples are given):

- Should the person be visited by a faith leader prior to death? For example, the Last Rites to the dying person is an important part of the Catholic tradition.
- Are there any specific people who should be with the person as they die?
- Who can/should care for the body after death? Muslim tradition dictates that the body should be cared for by family members of the same gender, while Traveller communities traditionally do not touch the dead and would request 'outsiders' to do this.
- Are there any time considerations? In the Jewish faith, for example, the body should be buried as soon as possible, while Buddhists believe that the body should not be touched for 3–8 hours after the last breath as the spirit is believed to linger.

Think about the area where you work, are there many faiths and traditions that are prevalent within the locality? Research which death rituals are relevant to this population.

It is important to remember that the death of someone that you have cared for can have an impact on you personally too. It may be that you have looked after them for some time or they may remind you of someone you know, for example, they may be a similar age or appearance or have similar mannerisms. It may be that you are with the person when they die, but more often than not, you will not be there. It is important, however, to know when someone that you have cared for has died, so it is useful to discuss with colleagues, or as a team, how you would like to share such information with each other. Is it right to call or text a colleague to let them know? Should the information wait until they are next at work? Some areas have a 'sign' if someone within the organisation has died. These are very subtle such as a snowflake decoration or a specific flower on the office window so that staff know and can enquire further. Deciding how best to relay such message is best discussed within your team.

Some hospices, hospitals, care homes will still talk of the person at handover the day(s) following the death. If possible they will avoid admitting anyone to that bed for a period of time after the death. This shows respect for the person who has died but also those caring for them.

Once a death has been registered, a funeral will be organised. This is an opportunity for people to pay their last respects and say good-bye. It may be that you feel that you want to attend. This is a personal choice. It may be that you want to support the family or it may be that it helps you to say goodbye to the person you have cared for. Always check first with the family if this is acceptable to them.

People grieve in different ways. You may choose to send a sympathy card to the family, either personally or on behalf of the organisation that cared for them – these can bring great comfort to the bereaved but also help the carer have a sense of 'closure'. It may also be appro-priate to mark the anniversary of the death. Care homes and hos-pices often keep a book of remembrance recording the date of death which is opened to the relevant page each year or a candle may be lit, some plant a shrub to honour the person. Families will often invite people who have cared for the person to attend the funeral, which, for some, may be appropriate. All of these are relatively simple but can be powerful ways of acknowledging that someone has died and celebrating their life.

Loss, grief and bereavement

> You don't know who is important to you until you actually lose them.
>
> (Mahatma Gandhi, 1869–1948)

Following the death of someone close to them, a person may have a variety of responses. Loss, grief and bereavement are a very personal experience. In the 1970s, Elizabeth Kübler-Ross proposed a model of bereavement, identifying key stages that the person may go through. The model has its critics and it should never be thought that someone will start at the top of the list and travel to the fifth stage in a straight line! The stages are not experienced by everyone and people may jump between them, however, the stages can be useful to consider how the bereaved person may feel:

1. *Denial* – finding it difficult to accept that the person has actually died.
2. *Anger* – a sense of abandonment that they have been left, anger perhaps that others still have their spouse/parent/friend.
3. *Bargaining* – 'the what if questions'.
4. *Depression* – lowness of mood as a direct response to the loss.
5. *Acceptance* – being able to say that they accept that the person has died and that they now will move on.

The people that we are caring for often die expectedly and at the end of a long illness or after increasing frailty. It can be a relief for a family when the person actually dies. While this time will be tinged with sadness, it is important that the bereaved family or friends can voice how they genuinely feel without fear of being judged.

Practical ways in which you can help someone who is bereaved

There are many leaflets, websites and organisations that can offer advice on helping someone who is bereaved. It is essential to remember that in the same way that every relationship is unique, so is every bereavement and each will take different courses. Listed below are some simple practical tips that may help:

- Encourage the person to talk about how they feel – they may express the emotions that we discussed above. They may be angry with the person for leaving them but in the same conversation accept that they had to die.
- Listen to them, give them space to talk but avoid saying 'I understand' because can we really?
- Offer practical help. This extract from a conversation with three children in their twenties whose mother died sums this up.

> The most helpful thing was the people who did simple things for us, things that we needed. They would come around with a casserole or pick up milk. We were very moved by a card that an older couple who knew Mum sent: it said, 'I can sew and my husband is good with paperwork – we would really love to help you if you think we can.' What was least helpful was when people said: 'What you need to do is …'

This practical help can also take the form of phone call, text message or call, just checking how things are going. Such messages can be particularly helpful at key times such as birthdays, anniversaries, etc. Sometimes it is important that the person feels that they have permission to feel how they are feeling. It's about saying, 'It's OK to feel sad' – that is very different from saying, 'I understand.'

Avoid asking, 'What can I do to help?' Though this may be said with a kind sentiment, we often hear that the bereaved person finds it difficult to respond. It is hard to concentrate and this is another thing for them to think about and come up with an answer. Try to offer them something that they can refuse or accept.

These simple things are practical ways in which we can help a friend, a colleague or a family member who has experienced loss. For some people, this will be sufficient but other people may need more in-depth support. People who die in the care of hospices, whether at home or in a hospice, will be offered bereavement support before and after the person dies. General practitioners can link people to professional counselling services and there are also many charities that can offer support, such as Cruse. There can, however, be waiting lists for these services.

What to do when someone dies and afterwards: things to remember

- After someone has died, make sure they look as cared for as possible so that relatives sitting with them can take comfort.
- Death must be verified (confirmed) before the body can be moved to the funeral directors. In the absence of a doctor, this can be done by a nurse who has undergone appropriate training.
- Only a doctor can certify a death (i.e. confirm cause of death). If a doctor is present, a death can be verified and certified at the same time.
- We must be sensitive to the cultural wishes of someone who passes away.

 It can be hard for you when someone you have been caring for dies, so in **Chapter 11** we will look at looking after yourself and your colleagues.

How can we look after ourselves?

Clair Sadler and Gill Thomas

Caring for people at the end of their life can be rewarding and enjoyable. It can, however, also be really tough and demanding, both emotionally and physically. The work can become increasingly stressful and the effects of this can sometimes 'sneak up' on us . We need to be clear about how to look after ourselves, why this is important, and what to do if we recognise we or our colleagues are struggling.

This chapter will explore:

- why it is important that we acknowledge the emotional strain of our work;
- how to identify when it is getting too demanding and difficult;
- ways that we can manage the demands;
- practical ideas and strategies that we can develop;
- top tips from the contributors of this book.

Throughout this book we have looked at the stories of Maria, Albert and Jenny, now we are going to look at the stories of three of the people who cared for them.

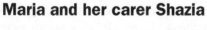

Maria and her carer Shazia

Shazia has been a carer for the last 18 months since her only child started school. She has a close family but things have been difficult with her ex-partner recently. Shazia has cared for Maria for 6 months – they have always had a warm and friendly relationship and love to 'chat', they are both big fans of soap operas and love to discuss what they have watched on

TV. Shazia has been on holiday and has not seen Maria for a couple of weeks. On her next visit, she sees a marked change in Maria's condition – she seems much more breathless, reluctant to get out of bed and seems very tired. Shazia feels worried and upset to see Maria looking so different as she has known her for such a long time. She says she just wants to go home and cry.

Albert and his carer Bob

Bob has looked after Albert for 6 months. The rest of the team at the care home have noticed that Bob does not quite seem himself over the last week or two since he came back from holiday and heard that Albert died. Bob had to ask the team leader what happened to Albert but no one told him. Bob always used to be cracking a joke with the residents and his mates but now he seems snappy and irritable. He says: 'I am just keeping my head down.'

Jenny and her carer Erika

Since Erika started working as a carer, she never had any sick leave but today she has not come to work. She has texted one of her colleagues to say that she has had enough of looking after people and cannot be bothered to come in, she said they 'owe' me a sick day. This really is out of character for her.

These three carers enjoyed their roles and got great satisfaction out of their work, but for each of them something happened that changed this. It is important that we are aware of the impact that looking after someone is having on us and on our colleagues, so that we can stop this work being 'too much'. If it becomes too much, there are signs that we can look for in ourselves and others. The end result, if we do not do something about these signs, is something called 'burnout'. Burnout can be described as long-term exhaustion alongside a reduced interest in work. For some people, this can mean that it becomes hard to switch off from work and separate work from home life. For some people, acknowledging that they are experiencing some of these signs may be sufficient; for others, they may need to take a short or extended break from their role. It is really important that we support our colleagues if we are aware of these signs and see them acting differently. It is also important that we have in place support structures so that we can (hopefully) avoid arriving at a point of burnout in the first place. The worst possible state that this can get to is when a person loses all sense of empathy and compassion for the people that they are looking after and become desensitised to them as ordinary people who need help. We sadly have all heard of some distressing stories when staff, in a variety of care settings, have become actively uncaring and possibly cruel, because they are so disengaged in their work and the people they are looking after.

What signs would lead you to believe that you or a colleague was starting to struggle with their role?

Setting boundaries

We said earlier in this book that if we are employed to look after someone, we need to keep a professional boundary and be sure of what our role is. The person that we are caring for often enjoys hearing about our lives, what we have been doing and about our family. We have to be careful, however, that we are not so open about ourselves that our work and our personal life become mixed together. It would not be appropriate to talk about our worries at work to the people we are looking after: they do not have to look after us. We may have shared interests with the people we care for but it would be equally inappropriate to meet with them or their familes outside the working day.

Dealing with burnout

Burnout is not simply a result of working long hours. It is more commonly a collection of different factors. Tiredness is often one of them but also the nature of the work that we do. Constantly caring can be demanding. Over a period of time, if there is no space or no one to talk to about the distressing things that we see, it can become increasingly hard to make sense of what we are experiencing and this can lead to burnout. This can look like depression and sadness. There can be a loss of energy or lethargy. It may be a disinterest and disconnect with the people that we care for and work with.

How do we recognise burnout?

It is really important that, if we have seen burnout in someone or in ourselves, that we do something so as to avoid facing the mental and or physical health problems that can ensue.

Recognition and acknowledgment are vital. This can be as simple as recognising the person is not their 'normal' self. They may become more irritable or easily annoyed, less responsive to emotional events, over-engaged with certain people that they are caring for or simply quieter. They may seem a bit low in mood or you may experience them being a bit lethargic or not being so keen to volunteer to do things that need doing.

Possible consequences of burnout

When the cost of caring becomes too high, this can have an obvious impact on the individual. The impact on the carer can include:

● health-related problems – stress, anxiety, depression, sleep disturbance, physical manifestations;
● family disruption – irritability and disharmony at home;
● reduced performance or commitment and also reduced satisfaction within their role.

Burnout can therefore also have a great impact on the person who the 'burnt out' person is caring for.

Building resilience (or the ability to bounce back)

> It is not the strongest of the species that survive, nor the most intelligent, but the one most responsive to change.
> (Charles Darwin, 1809–1882)

When we are looking after people who are approaching the end of their lives, the reality is that they are going to die. We therefore can meet and get to know over time many people who will be in our care. We will be building new relationships again and again and inevitably we will experience multiple losses. Building resilience is about being able to sustain ourselves and learn how to feel compassion while holding onto the professional boundary that stops work from eating us up and spitting us out. If we have looked after someone for a long time, we will experience a sense of loss. If your working pattern is shifts, it can be really hard coming back to work a few days after someone has died and finding a new person in their room or bed. The rest of the team has had a bit of time to get used to this death whereas you have just walked into this dramatic change.

Psychologists say that we can actively do things to build up our resilience to this work, and here are some of the things that can really help. Some of the things that can help build a sense of well-being and a work–life balance are:

- *Connecting* – develop and have good social networks outside work, friends you can talk to and get involved in some fun social activities.
- *Being active* – dance, walk, ride a bike, discover some physical activity that suits your level of fitness and mobility.
- *Taking notice* – begin to be mindful of your everyday life, e.g. really notice some small detail about your journey to work. Introduce some **mindfulness** practice which will be discussed later in this chapter.
- *Keep learning* – sign up for a course, have a go at that instrument you used to play, or offer to take on a new responsibility at work. Learning something new can build your confidence.
- *Group membership* – we can get support from like-minded people and spending time with them. This can take many forms: a quiz team, zumba class or faith group perhaps.
- *Give back* – do something nice for a friend or even a stranger. Smile at someone you do not know. Look out to what is happening in your local community. Get involved and support a charitable event.

When we feel happy about what we are involved with away from work this will naturally build up our resilience bank, which we need to keep an eye on when we are working in this area of care.

What may help?

- *Offloading* to a friend or colleague.
- *Acknowledgement* that the role can be demanding is important and strategies can be put in place to address this. Awareness of

possible signs in ourselves or others is vital. It often takes some-one else to point out how drained we are becoming for us to acknowledge this. Things that may help can be formal or infor-mal. Many employers offer formal support for staff. This is often done through a helpline offering a confidential counselling service.

- *Reflection* on a recent situation with a colleague or colleagues can also be helpful. Remember it can be equally useful to reflect on situations that went well as those that went badly or were challenging. This could also happen with the team after some-one has died or if there is a particularly challenging situation that occurs or is ongoing.
- *Time out* is vital and most employers will encourage staff to have regular holidays away from their role. There can be a temptation for some to work extended hours or take on addi-tional work.
- *Clinical supervision* is something that is now expected to occur for most healthcare professionals. This is a regularly planned and protected time once every four to six weeks to reflect on the emotional impact of working with people. It is a good time to also celebrate what has gone well so that we can learn from this. A clinical supervisor is not normally your line manager so that it can be a confidential time to reflect in an honest way on the work you have been doing and its impact on you. It has good outcomes for employers too in that it is often seen as a very positive thing for employers to offer this and it can help with staff retention and recruitment.

There are other techniques that can really help us on a daily basis and here are some that you might find useful.

Mindfulness

Mindfulness is an increasingly popular practice which is a way of taking a moment to pause and just be 'still'and taking a little time out in our hectic lives, to have a clear mind that is not a mind full of feel-ing or worry. We can spend so much time fretting about what has happened or worrying about what could happen that it is often diffi-cult to stop and just be still.

These are two quick mindfulness exercises. Both take a very short amount of concentrated time and may help you to re-focus.

Two minute exercise

Find somewhere where you can see a wall clock or a watch with a second hand. Spend a minute watching the second hand marking a minute. Having watched that minute of time pass, now focus on your breathing for a full minute. Notice how your breath feels as you breathe in, or as you breathe out. Does it feel warm, does it feel cool? Where else do you feel the breath in your body? Really focus all your attention on your breath.

Breath and feet

Find somewhere that you can sit down. Focus all your attention down to your feet. If you feel comfortable having your eyes closed, all the better. Really think about your feet, how do they feel? Where is your weight? Is it in your toes or the soles of your feet? What temperature are they? How does it feel to have all your attention in your feet? Does this feel like you might be having a different relationship with your feet? So keeping your attention down in your feet, now focus on your breathing, notice how your breath feels as you breathe in, or as you breathe out, does it feel warm? Does it feel cool? Where else do you feel the breath in your body? Really focus all your attention on your breath. After a couple of minutes, bring yourself back to the room and open your eyes.

These are two very simple exercises that you can initiate into your day. As with anything, the more practice, the more natural it will become. This is something you can do for yourself; your employer may also have services in place that could help you. Some have confidential help lines, others a buddy service, for example.

Reflective groups

Caring for someone and supporting their family can at times be challenging and distressing. It is therefore important that with the team that you work you can feel supported when things are getting tough or upsetting. Times for the team to offload and share these challenges are really important and can be achieved through a reflective group. A reflective group can be set up to allow this to happen. The formality can vary depending on the group and members but certain ground rules should be considered.

- Someone is asked to facilitate the group, ideally someone who has not been directly involved.
- A time is agreed, which means as many of the team can attend, or the session is repeated.
- A room is booked where there will be no interruptions.
- Everyone has time to speak and voice what they are thinking or feeling.

Each person needs to have time to tell their version of how they have felt challenged. They will also hear the experiences of others and possibly fill in gaps in the story. The person leading the group needs to be aware of the time and make sure that each person has spoken if they wish to.

Reflective groups allow a team to share challenges, and help team members support each other and feel supported themselves as they do not feel alone in having these experiences. These groups can help with staff morale, sickness levels and retention of staff, therefore are a highly valuable investment in a team.

Find out what kind of formal support is available to you from your employer.

There are many informal ways that may help, such as exercise, time to relax, time on own – walking, reading or being with family and friends.

What formal and informal things do you think would help you cope with your role?

All the contributors to this book work in palliative care. They have identified some of the things that help them. Read them and ask yourself – would any of these work for me? What would I need to do to make it happen?

> For my self-care, I love supervision! I use formal and informal supervision and colleagues to reflect on situations and individuals that 'stay with us'. For me, talking it through with others helps me to understand why I am experiencing these feelings. It helps me remember the enormity of some of the situations we work in and how my feelings and values influence my work. By recognising these feelings, it helps me to maintain boundaries and manage them so that it does not impair my ability to assess a situation critically.
>
> (Sarah, social worker, Chapter 7)

> I try to take regular holidays, at least once every three months. I try not to get over-tired and have a regular holistic treatment about once every six weeks. Confide and share with my colleagues when things are tough and listen to their wisdom.
>
> (Roz, staff nurse, Chapter 8)

> I am very aware of the need to be able to switch off from work so that is the first thing I do. I have handed over to the next team and as I walk out, I leave work at work. Obviously clinical supervision helps and I also have a spiritual director. I swim regularly and I like relaxation touch therapies such as reflexology, which are really helpful.
>
> (Irene, staff nurse, Chapter 8)

> Ensuring you access peer support and debrief after difficult situations. Ensure when home life starts to impact on work or vice versa, that you access supervision to explore how to manage this. Be open and honest. This at times is an upsetting job so do not do it alone – access support from the team. I love to socialise with family and friends.
>
> (Hayley, social worker, Chapter 7)

> Other than the wine, I look after myself by cycling home so that by the time I have cycled up the hills on the way home, I have forgotten the stresses of work. Also I value my friends who make me laugh.
>
> (Amanda, doctor, Chapter 4)

On my way home in the car, I often sing very loudly to anything on the radio. My route home means that I cross the River Thames by one of the road bridges. I say to myself I will think about work until I have crossed the river. Sometimes I will drive the long way home so I can let things go for the day. I walk regularly and sing in a choir.

(Gill, art therapist, Chapter 4)

One of the main ways I support myself is by clinical supervision. I find having someone I trust and respect who listens, encourages and challenges me, is supportive. I have learnt to value balance in my life. All work and no play is not healthy. I need to ensure I make time for all the different aspects of my life. That means giving myself permission to relax and receive care as well as give care. Just as we care for our patients', mind, body and spirit, I too need to nourish my mind, body and spirit. Another important source of support is the friendship of my colleagues. Other nurses understand the pressures and strains of the work and they are there for me whether we are laughing or crying, and sometimes doing both at the same moment!

(Helen, staff nurse, Chapter 8)

As you take off your uniform (or work clothes), consciously think that your uniform is your day and take it off. Your day clothes now represent life outside of work. As you walk out the door of your workplace, think consciously about leaving the day behind. You may want to talk about your day with a colleague, team member or manager before you leave.

(Liz, research lead, Chapter 2)

The hospice has strategies to help people cope, but I find the support of our colleagues helps as much as anything.

(Christine, staff nurse, Chapter 5)

Think back to Bob, Shazia and Erika, the carers whom we met at the beginning of this chapter. If you were their colleague, what would you suggest or do to help?

Looking after you: things to remember

Caring for people at the end of their life can be both satisfying and rewarding. It is important to realise that at times we will find the work difficult – for whatever reason. We need to pre-empt this and think about what support we need and how we can get it:

- Consider the impact on you of long-term caring.
- Set up your own support strategies.
- Look out for your colleagues.
- Discuss with your line manager what resources are available to you.

Frequently asked questions

This book has given you an overview of how best to look after someone who is dying. You may still have some questions and this chapter offers answers to some these frequently asked questions.

Question: Does the person have to pay for specialist equipment?

Answer: Generally, no, essentials such as bed, mattress, wheelchairs and similar aids are free of charge. Stair lifts and other major adaptations would not be included.

Question: What is the difference between a Macmillan nurse and a hospice clinical nurse specialist (CNS), or a clinical nurse specialist in palliative care?

Answer: Fundamentally there is no difference. All offer a similar service. The main difference is funding in that hospice clinical nurse specialists are employed by a hospital or hospice, whereas Macmillan nurses are employed by the charity Macmillan Cancer Care. Who the care is offered by is often dependent on the area where the person is being cared for.

Question: Why doesn't everyone who is dying get specialist palliative or hospice care?

Answer: The simple answer is because not everyone needs it. People can be well supported with minimal or no involvement from specialist services which frees up the services to focus on those people who do have complex care needs.

Question: What happens if someone has an advance care plan and then changes their minds?

Answer: It is not uncommon for people to change their minds as circumstances and experiences change, and as long as they have mental capacity, they can change their plan at any time, either in writing or by telling people such as their family and the people caring for them. The changes should be recorded in the person's relevant notes or records. If a solicitor has been involved in writing any of the planning documents, they should also be informed.

Question: Can a family say that they do not want their relative to be resuscitated?

Answer: We would hope that any decision like this would be made together with a family but, fundamentally, it is the choice of the person. The exception to this would be in situations where the person was deemed not to have capacity to make their own decisions. In this case, it is the responsibility of the doctor to decide on the basis of 'best interest'. In making the decision, the doctor will take into account the family wishes, what (if anything) is known about the person's wishes, the person's physical condition and also the possibility of resuscitation being successful. In most cases of expected death, the person's body has already been weakened through their illness so the possibility of a resuscitation attempt being successful is extremely low.

Question: Will the clinical nurse specialist or Macmillan nurse visit someone who is dying every day?

Answer: This will depend on the person's needs. Some people do not require any specialist care, others require a lot more. For many, it can be that contact is made and advice given. It will also depend on the way services are organised in the area the person lives. The CNS/ Macmillan nurse rarely provides hands-on care, rather advice, support and guidance.

Question: Do all people die in pain?

Answer: This is a very real fear for a lot of people approaching the end of their life. However, many people do not have pain and for those who do, there are lots of ways which pain can be improved. The GP and district nurse may well be able to help with most types of pain but can involve the specialists to help if needed.

Question: Can someone die without a syringe pump?

Answer: Most certainly. Syringe pumps are the exception rather than the rule. Some people do not require any medication to manage their symptoms, others are able to continue to take medicine by another route until they die, for example, by mouth or patch.

Question: Are dying people disturbed by noise?

Answer: Sometimes we think that because someone is dying, the room, and everyone around the person, should be kept quiet – this is not the case. Be watchful that the person is not distressed by noise but, generally, if they have been used to having the TV on in the background, music playing or the noise of children playing outside an open window, that does not need to change.

Question: Are general care plans and advance care plans the same thing?

Answer: No, a general care plan is the plan for the person's current and continuing social and health care needs. An advance care plan considers what a person would like as they approach the end of their life.

Question: Do you have to pay for hospice care?

Answer: No. There is no charge. The majority of hospices are independent and funded mainly through charitable donations with only a small part of their income coming from the NHS. There are a small number of hospices who are actually part of the NHS.

Glossary

In this Glossary, you will find words and abbreviations that are often used in end of life care. Some will have been used in this book, others you may be more or less familiar with. As you come across words or phrases, jot them down, find their meaning and start your own list!

Abbey pain scale Widely used assessment tool for the measurement of pain in people who cannot verbalise, e.g. people with dementia.

Adjuvant A drug given with another drug to increase its effect.

Advance care planning (ACP) Advance care planning is a process of discussion and reflection about goals, values and preferences for future treatment in the context of an anticipated deterioration in the patient's condition with loss of capacity to make decisions and communicate these to others.

Advance decision or advance directive A statement of a patient's wish to refuse a particular type of medical treatment or care if they become unable to make or communicate decisions for themselves.

Advance statement A statement made by someone that outlines how they would or would not wish to be cared for if they became incapable of expressing this. Usually the statement relates to place of care and cultural or religious preferences but may also relate to statements regarding treatment preferences.

Aroma stone An electric diffuser that gently warms aromatherapy oils to scent the surrounding atmosphere which can help remove unpleasant smells. Aromatherapy oils may also reduce the feeling of sickness and help a person to relax. Aroma stones are safer than using candles or burners.

Breakthrough pain Transient background pain in otherwise managed pain.

Care plan This is sometimes referred to as a 'general care plan'. A written document jointly agreed by the patient and professional. It is the tangible record of the process of care. It should allow a holistic approach to care, empowering individuals to bring all relevant areas of their life to the discussion. It can also help in the audit of service delivery.

Clinical supervision Regular planned and protected time, once every four to six weeks, where an individual or a group will meet with a supervisor to reflect on issues relating to their role.

Complementary therapies A treatment given alongside other conventional methods of medical management, such as massage and hypnotherapy.

Coordinate My Care Coordinate My Care is an electronic record management system that can be accessed by the multiprofessional team so that everyone is aware of the person's end of life care needs and wishes.

DNACPR Abbreviation of 'Do Not Attempt Cardiopulmonary Resuscitation'. See Chapter 2 for a discussion of this.

Dossette box Sometimes known as a pill organiser. A box that is pre-loaded by the patient, family member or pharmacist. The box is divided into compartments by days of the week and usually by times of the day and the correct amount of medication placed in each compartment.

End of life care An important part of palliative care, and usually refers to the care of a person during the last phase of their life.

End stage The final period or phase in the course of a progressive disease leading to a patient's death.

Fatigue A feeling of becoming tired easily, being unable to complete usual activity, feeling weak and having difficulty concentrating, which is often disease-related.

Hospice care Care of a person as an inpatient, using day services or in the community, that focuses on the management of symptoms and needs of chronically ill, seriously ill or terminally ill people. The focus is on holistic care meeting physical, social, psychological and spiritual needs.

Illness trajectory Path or route followed by a certain illness.

Key worker A key worker is a healthcare or care professional who, with the patient's consent, takes the lead in coordinating the patient's care. The key worker also acts as the main point of contact for the patient, their carer and all the professionals who are involved in their care.

Lasting power of attorney (LPA) A lasting power of attorney allows the person to appoint others to make decisions on their behalf. This is a legally binding document for people who envisage a time ahead when they may be unable to manage their personal and legal affairs or health and welfare needs.

Life-limiting Illness that is known to shorten a person's life such as heart, kidney or liver failure, diabetes, lung disease, motor neurone disease or multiple sclerosis.

Life-threatening Illness that carries a strong probability the person will die as a result of it.

Medical certificate of cause of death (MCCD) Document confirming the cause of a person's death. Completed by the person's doctor usually within 24 hours of the death.

Mindfulness A technique to help focus and become more aware of the present moment by focusing on feelings and sensations such as breathing.

Multiprofessional team Group of professionals from different healthcare backgrounds who work together to offer coordinated care to a person.

Nebuliser Means of administering medication as a mist which can be inhaled.

NHS continuing healthcare NHS continuing healthcare is free care outside of hospital that is arranged and funded by the NHS. It is only available for people who need ongoing healthcare and meet the eligibility criteria. To be eligible for NHS continuing healthcare, the person must be assessed as having a 'primary health need' and have a complex medical condition and substantial and ongoing care needs.

Occupational therapist Healthcare professional whose focus is on optimising a person's independent functioning.

Opioids Pain-relieving medication, e.g. morphine, codeine.

Palliative care Palliative care is the active holistic care of patients with advanced progressive illness. Management of pain and other symptoms and provision of psychological, social and spiritual support are paramount. The goal of palliative care is the achievement of the best quality of life for patients and their families. Many aspects of palliative care are also applicable earlier in the course of the illness in conjunction with other treatments (Source: NCPC).

Person-centred care Care based on the goals of the individual receiving the care, the person being seen as an equal partner in health care.

Pressure sores Also known as bedsores, pressure ulcers and decubitus ulcers. Wounds that develop as a result of constant pressure or friction on one area, often the heels or sacrum but can occur anywhere.

Primary health need Presence of illness that is progressing and requires continuing support due to its severity and unpredictability which will demonstrate the need for continuing healthcare funding.

Profiling bed Also often referred to as a 'hospital bed', it is an electronically operated bed whereby sections of the bed can be moved or profiled (e.g. raising the head) so that the person can be moved easily into a range of positions. The height of the bed can also be adjusted to help with moving and handling of the person.

Respite care Short or temporary care to offer relief to family members. This may be planned or as a reaction to a crisis.

Rigor mortis Rigor mortis is when the body naturally becomes stiffened after death, triggered by chemical changes.

Specialist palliative care Specialist palliative care encompasses hospice care (including inpatient hospice, day hospice services, hospice at home) as well as a range of other specialist advice, support and care such as that provided by hospital palliative care teams. Specialist palliative care should be available on the basis of need, not diagnosis.

Supportive care Care that helps people approaching the end of life, and their families and carers, to cope with the symptoms and treatments of their disease as well as their psychological, social and spiritual needs. It helps the patient to maximise the benefits of treatment and to live as well as possible with the effects of the disease.

Surprise question A question posed by healthcare professional as to whether the person that they are caring for is approaching the end of their life. 'Would you be surprised if this person died in the next 12 months?'

Symptom A change in the body or mind experienced by a person indicating a disease or other disorders. In this book we have divided this into physical and non-physical symptoms (see Chapters 5 and 6).

Syringe pump A syringe pump is a small portable battery-operated pump which drives the plunger of a syringe at an accurately controlled rate to deliver drugs. Syringe pumps provide symptom control via a continuous subcutaneous infusion of drugs to treat pain and other distressing symptoms when other routes are inappropriate or ineffective.

Terminal care Refers to care provided in the hours or days preceding death.

Total pain 'Total pain' describes the physical, mental, social and spiritual components to distress and suffering in terminally ill cancer patients (Saunders 1978).

Verification of expected death (VOED) Following training, a nurse or paramedic can verify that a person has died and completes a VOED form. The death will still need to be certified by a doctor but it means that the family can be informed, clinical paraphernalia can be removed and a funeral director can be contacted once the death has been verified.

Waterlow scale A nationally recognised tool to assess a person's risk of developing a pressure ulcer.

Appendix: Useful websites, books and other resources

The chapters in this book have looked at the key areas of caring for someone who is dying. Additional resources that you may wish to access can be found below and in the references section that follows at the end of the book. Please remember that websites, their addresses and content do change, but these are correct at the time of going to press. The sites listed are well established and considered reputable.

Books aimed at children

A number of books are available to help people who have experienced the loss of someone close to them. A few of these are listed below together with the age for which they are recommended.

For age 4 and up

Keller, H. (1987) *Good-Bye Max*. London: Julia MacRae.

Thomas , P. (2001) *I Miss You: A First Look at Death*. London: Hodder Wayland.

For 5–8 years

Durant, A. (2013) *Always and Forever*. Oxford: Random House.

Ironside, V. (1996) *The Huge Bag of Worries*. Hove: Macdonald Young.

Varley, S. (2013) *Badger's Parting Gifts*. London: Andersen.

For 9–12 years

Mellonie, B. and Ingpen, R. (1983) *Beginnings and Endings with Lifetimes in Between*. Lumpsfield: Paper Tiger.

Rosen, M. (2004) *Michael Rosen's Sad Book*. London: Walker Books.

Wilson J. (2001) *The Cat Mummy*. London: Doubleday.

For 13–16 years

Grollman, E. (1993) *Straight Talk about Death for Teenagers*. Boston: Beacon Press.

Lloyd, C. (1989) *The Charlie Barber Treatment*. London: Walker Books.

Wilson, J. (1995) *Double Act*. London: Corgi Yearling.

Websites

BBC and Beliefnet

There is a vast amount of online information about the different faith systems but, as each person's relationship with religion is different, it is important not to impose religious rites and rituals onto individuals without first discussing it with those concerned. However, some prior knowledge can be useful and the BBC provides a reliable source of information about the major religions and beliefnet.com has published a useful summary of transition rituals by faith.

http://www.bbc.co.uk/religion/religions/ (accessed Oct. 2014).

http://www.beliefnet.com/Health/Health-Support/Grief-and-Loss/2001/05/Transition-Rituals.aspx (accessed Oct. 2014).

Dying Matters

www.dyingmatters.org

Dying Matters is a coalition of organisations and individuals which aims to help people talk more openly about dying, death and bereavement, and to make plans for the end of life. The website is regularly updated with campaigns, stories, advice and suggestions.

GOV.UK

www.gov.uk

GOV.UK is the gateway to government services and information and provides comprehensive information on benefits and a practical guide to the process of registering a death.

McKinley T34 training

http://www.cmemedical.co.uk/online-training/

T34 is an ambulatory syringe pump that is used to administer continuous medication in both inpatient and outpatient settings. The manufacturer of the pumps offers useful online training material and guidance on the use of the pumps on their website.

National Council for Palliative Care (NCPC)

www.ncpc.org.uk

The NCPC is the umbrella charity for organisations and individuals involved in palliative, end of life and hospice care in England, Wales and Northern Ireland.

NHS Choices

www.nhs.uk

The NHS Choices website provides accredited and up-to-date information on conditions and treatment, symptoms, social and healthcare services, and information on which benefits are available.

The Scottish Partnership for Palliative Care

www.palliativecarescotland.org.uk

The Scottish Partnership for Palliative Care is the NCPC's sister organisation offering services in Scotland.

World Health Organization (WHO)

www.who.int

WHO is the United Nations authority on health matters, research, standards, policy trends and technical support. If you search on 'palliative care' on the website, a global resource of information is returned.

Charities

Age UK

www.ageuk.org.uk

Age UK is a large national charity offering advice and support to older people. They have a number of publications and campaigns but *When Someone Dies: A Step-By-Step Guide to What to Do* may be of particular help.

Bereavement Advice Centre

www.bereavementadvice.org

The Bereavement Advice Centre provide a helpful leaflet, which can be downloaded from the website, entitled 'What to do when someone dies: a practical guide'.

Carers Trust

www.carers.org

The Carers Trust works to support those involved as unpaid carers of relatives and friends. The charity provides information, advice, respite and education.

Child Bereavement UK

www.childbereavement.org.uk

Child Bereavement UK supports families and educates professionals when a child dies or is dying, or when a child is facing bereavement. The following two items in this section may also prove useful in the case of child grief or child bereavement, as well as Winston's Wish at the end of this list.

Citizens Advice Bureau

www.citizensadvicebureau.org.uk

The Citizens Advice Bureau provides free, independent, confidential and impartial advice to everyone on their rights and responsibilities.

Cruse Bereavement Care

www.cruse.org.uk

Cruse Bereavement Care is a charity which supports someone after the death of someone close to them. Face-to-face and group support are delivered by trained bereavement support volunteers across the UK and information, publications and support for children are also available.

Grief Encounter

www.griefencounter.org.uk

The charity helps families address difficult issues such as death and provides free access to support services. There are also many locally run support services targeted towards children, such as riprap, www.riprap.org.uk, a support service for children whose parent has been diagnosed with cancer, and SeeSaw, www.seesaw.org.uk, which provides grief support to children and young children.

Help the Hospices

www.helpthehospices.org.uk

While the focus of this book has not been on hospice care, hospices may play a part in the care of someone you are looking after. This is a charity for hospice care in the UK, providing information and support to anyone interested in hospice care.

Maggie's Centres

www.maggiescentres.org.uk

Maggie's Centres are mainly linked to cancer centres around the country. They offer free practical, emotional and social support to people with cancer and their families and friends. Help is offered freely to anyone with any type of cancer.

Macmillan Cancer Support

www.macmillan.org.uk

Macmillan is a large national cancer charity offering practical, medical and financial support to people with cancer and those who care for them.

Pets as Therapy

www.petsastherapy.org

Pets as Therapy is a national community-based charity providing therapeutic visits to hospitals, hospices, nursing and care homes, special needs schools and a variety of other establishments from volunteers with their pet dogs and cats.

The Social Care Institute for Excellence (SCIE)

www.SCIE.org.uk

The SCIE is an independent charity that works to improve care services in the UK by sharing knowledge about what works.

Winston's Wish

www.winstonswish.org.uk

Winston's Wish is the leading childhood bereavement charity in the UK. They offer practical support and guidance to bereaved children, their families and professionals.

Useful resources for nurses

Royal College of Nursing (RCN)

www.rcn.org.uk

The RCN is the UK's largest nursing union and provides support to its members, along with professional development and information on news and events critical to the nursing profession.

Resources and DVDs

Naomi Feil (2009). Gladys Wilson and Naomi Feil. [Online]. USA: Memory Bridge. https://www.youtube.com/watch?v=CrZXz10FcVM (accessed Oct-14). This is the moving encounter between a therapist and a woman, Naomi, who has advanced dementia.

What Do You See (2005). [Film]. Amanda Waring. dir. UK: Looking for Magic. *What Do You See* is a moving film following a day in the life of a person having had a stroke. It offers insight into the need for compassionate care.

I Am Breathing (2013). [Film]. Emma Davie, dir. UK: Scottish Documentary Institute. *I Am Breathing* is a powerful documentary DVD following the life of a young man with motor neurone disease (MND) and his subsequent death.

References

Age UK (2014) *Care in Crisis*. London: Age UK. Available at: http://
www.ageuk.org.uk/Documents/EN-GB/Campaigns/CIC/Care_
in_Crisis_report_2014.pdf?epslanguage=en-GB?dtrk%3dtrue
(accessed Oct. 2014).

Department of Health (2008) *End of Life Care Strategy: Promoting
High Quality Care for Adults at the End of Their Life.* London:
TSO.

Available at: https://www.gov.uk/government/publications/end-of-
life-care-strategy-promoting-high-quality-care-for-adults-at-the-
end-of-their-life (accessed Oct. 2014).

Kübler-Ross, E. (1973) *On Death and Dying.* London: Tavistock.

Lunney, J. et al. (2003) Patterns of functional decline at the end of
life. *JAMA: The Journal of the American Medical Association,*
289(18): 2387–92.

Marie Curie (2012) *The Key Worker and the End of Life.* London:
Marie Curie Cancer Care. Available at: http://www.mariecurie.
org.uk/Documents/Commissioners-and-referrers/service-design/
Key-worker-leaflet-for-professionals.pdf (accessed Nov. 2014).

Murray, S.A. et al. (2005) Illness trajectories and palliative care. *BMJ,*
330: 1007–11.

The National Council for Palliative Care (2008) *The Mental Capacity
Act in Practice (2008): Guidance for End of Life Care.* London:
The National Council for Palliative Care.

The National Council for Palliative Care (2011) *Commissioning End
of Life Care: Initial Actions for New Commissioners.* London:
The National Council for Palliative Care. Available at: http://
www.ncpc.org.uk/sites/default/files/AandE.pdf (accessed Oct.
2014).

National Health Service (2008) End of Life Care Programme. *Advance
Care Planning: A Guide for Health and Social Care Staff.*

2nd edition. Leicester: National Health Service. Available at: http://beta.scie-socialcareonline.org.uk/advance-care-planning-a-guide-for-health-and-social-care-staff/r/a11G00000017ztAIAQ (accessed Oct. 2014).

Saunders C. (1989) Pain and impending death. In P.D. Wall and R. Melzak (eds) *Textbook of Pain*. 2nd edition. Edinburgh: Churchill Livingstone, pp. 624–31.

Stickley, T. (2011) From SOLER to SURETY for effective non-verbal communication. *Nurse Education in Practice*, 11(6): 395–8.

Who (World Health Organization) Available at: http://www.who.int/cancer/palliative/definition/en/ (accessed 7 April 2015).

Index

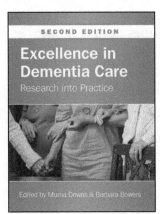

Excellence in Dementia Care
Principles and Practices
Second Edition

Downs and Bowers

ISBN: 9780335245338 (Paperback)
eBook: 9780335245345
2014

This scholarly yet accessible textbook is the most comprehensive single text in the field of dementia care. Drawn from research evidence, international expertise and good practice guidelines, the book has been crafted alongside people with dementia and their families. Case studies and quotes in every chapter illustrate the realities of living with dementia and bring the theory to life.

Key topics include:

- Dementia friendly communities
- Representations of dementia in the media
- Younger people with dementia
- The arts and dementia
- Whole person assessment
- Dementia friendly physical design
- Transitions in care
- Enhancing relationships between families and those with dementia

www.openup.co.uk

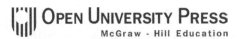

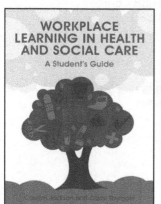

WORKPLACE LEARNING IN HEALTH AND SOCIAL CARE
A Student's Guide

Carolyn Jackson and Claire Thurgate

ISBN: 9780335237500 (Paperback)
eBook: 9780335239771
2011

This is a practical resource for anyone undertaking work based learning in health and social care. It introduces and explores the practicalities of learning in a healthcare setting, and is designed to help you make the most of your work based learning experience when studying for a foundation degree or other qualification.

Key features:

- Contains examples, vignettes and quotes
- Includes practical tools and worksheets to use in practice and study
- Provides practical strategies and exercises to strengthen capacity to learn at work and reflect on personal and professional development goals

www.openup.co.uk

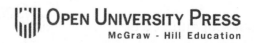

OPEN UNIVERSITY PRESS
McGraw - Hill Education

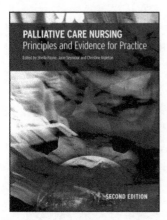

Palliative Care Nursing
Second Edition

Payne, Seymour and Ingleton

ISBN: 9780335221813 (Paperback)
eBook: 9780335236466
2008

The second edition of this innovative textbook has been extensively revised and updated to reflect new global developments in palliative care. This textbook reviews current research and examines the evidence base for palliative care policy and practice.

Key features include:

- What happens to people as they become ill
- How individuals cope as they near death and are dying
- How families and friends deal with bereavement and loss

www.openup.co.uk

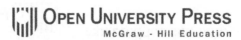

OPEN UNIVERSITY PRESS
McGraw - Hill Education

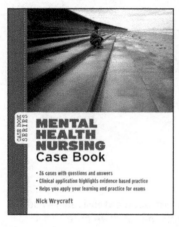

MENTAL HEALTH NURSING CASE BOOK

Nick Wrycraft

9780335242955 (Paperback)
September 2012

eBook also available

This case book is aimed at mental health nursing students and those going into mental health settings, such as social workers. The cases include a wide range of mental health diagnoses from common problems such as anxiety or depression through to severe and enduring conditions such as schizophrenia. The cases will be organised into sections by life stage from childhood through to old age.

Key features:

- Uses a case study approach which provides a realistic context that students will find familiar
- Each case study will commence with a practice focused scenario
- Provides a commentary offering insights, perspectives and references to theories, research and further explanations and discussion

www.openup.co.uk

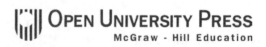